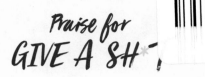

Praise for
GIVE A SH*T

"I love Ashlee's honest and fun writing style. It's so refreshing to read the truth about topics people like to pretend don't exist. Big fan!"

—Daniella Monet, actress and activist

"Become the superstar human you kind of knew you were but needed guidance on becoming . . . read this book and you (and the whole, wide world) will be better for it."

—Kathy Freston, *New York Times* bestselling author of *The Lean*, *Veganist*, and *Clean Protein*

"Saving the world can seem like a pretty daunting feat without a guidebook to start you on the right path. This is that book. Ashlee Piper gives you all the inspiration, information, and instruction you need to make those small changes that can have a huge impact."

—Annie Shannon, bestselling author of *Betty Goes Vegan* and *Mastering the Art of Vegan Cooking*

"A smart, quick, useful, and, yes, hilariously profane guide to living in ways that will make the world a far better place. Who knew being good could be so much fun?"

—Suzy Welch, *New York Times* bestselling author of *10-10-10* and co-author of *The Real-Life MBA*

"*Give a Sh*t* is like having every savvy article on going green— from how to properly recycle to tips on creating a non-toxic beauty routine—all in one place. It's the perfect dose of eco-guidance for anyone craving real, no-BS advice."

—Greta Eagan, author of *Wear No Evil: How to Change the World with Your Wardrobe*

"This is the guide well-intentioned-but-overwhelmed people have been waiting for. Thoughtful, funny, and utterly practical."

—Natalie Slater, author of
Bake and Destroy: Good Food for Bad Vegans

"Ashlee makes a strong case that it's not so hard to give a shit. She makes it chic to be eco-friendly for a new generation of consumers who don't want to choose between efficacy and sustainability. This book is so on point!"

—Leila Janah, CEO and founder, Samasource and LXMI and
author of *Give Work: Reversing Poverty One Job at a Time*

"Ashlee Piper is a maven of consciousness, a conduit to kindness, and a green glamazon of the highest order. She preaches the ethos I've been espousing for decades: you can look like a fox and still be truly good to the planet and all its inhabitants. This is a book all sustainable-curious, committed plant-eaters, and green fashionistas should have handy."

—Chloé Jo Davis,
founder/editor of GirlieGirlArmy

"Fun, friendly, and girl-powered (but dishing out the skinny on some serious stuff), this book will chat its way into your heart and, more importantly, into your choices. Piper's plan for saving animals and the planet also has you spiffing your style and living to the fullest."

—Victoria Moran,
author of *Main Street Vegan* and *Living a Charmed Life*

"Ashlee makes it easy to give a shit. This book is a simple, modern conversation with simple actionable plans to live by and really make a difference. None of us can afford to just suck air and take this life for granted. I think everyone needs a copy of this book!"

—Brook Harvey-Taylor, founder of Pacifica

GIVE A SH*T

Do Good. Live Better.
Save the Planet.

A PRACTICAL HANDBOOK BY
ASHLEE PIPER

RUNNING PRESS
PHILADELPHIA

Copyright © 2018 by Ashlee Piper
Illustrations copyright © 2018 by Paige Vickers except where noted.

Hachette Book Group supports the right to free expression and the value of copyright. The purpose of copyright is to encourage writers and artists to produce the creative works that enrich our culture.

The scanning, uploading, and distribution of this book without permission is a theft of the author's intellectual property. If you would like permission to use material from the book (other than for review purposes), please contact permissions@hbgusa.com. Thank you for your support of the author's rights.

Running Press
Hachette Book Group
1290 Avenue of the Americas, New York, NY 10104
www.runningpress.com
@Running_Press

Printed in Canada

First Edition: June 2018

Published by Running Press, an imprint of Perseus Books, LLC, a subsidiary of Hachette Book Group, Inc. The Running Press name and logo is a trademark of the Hachette Book Group.

The Hachette Speakers Bureau provides a wide range of authors for speaking events. To find out more, go to www.hachettespeakersbureau.com or call (866) 376-6591.

The publisher is not responsible for websites (or their content) that are not owned by the publisher.

Print book cover and interior design by Frances J. Soo Ping Chow
Illustrations: pages 15, 20, 30, 38, 41, 42, 46, 49, 55, 58, 68, 71, 72, 79, 90, 96, 136, 154, 158, 165, 170, 173, 186, 215, 219, 222, 227, 238 by GettyImages/Natasha_Pankina; pages 106–109 by GettyImages/Kittisak_Taramas; page 63 by GettyImages/kyuree

Library of Congress Control Number: 2017961282

ISBNs: 978-0-7624-6448-7 (paperback), 978-0-7624-6449-4 (ebook)

FRI

10 9 8 7 6 5 4 3 2 1

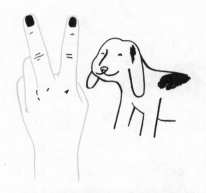

MOM FOR THE COMPASSION.

DAD FOR THE COURAGE.

BANJO FOR THE PURPOSE.

Contents

Introduction

How to Give a Shit

> "We are the ones
> we have been waiting for."
>
> —ALICE WALKER

I like to believe humanity is composed of pretty well-intentioned folks. We have a hunch that, no shit, the planet is dying under the weight of industrialized consumption and disposable culture and that we might have a little something to do with that. So we recycle our hearts out, buy fancy organic produce when it's on sale, and carry our colorful reusable water bottles to the gym (when we remember), all in the hopes of making a dent in an issue that's fast approaching DEFCON 1. But in a day and age when people claim to care increasingly more about sustainability, our planet is also in the worst state it's been in, well, ever (we'll get to specifics on that in a sec).[1] How can this be? Well, here's my hunch: the dissonance between our desire to be green and our sloth-like inaction stems from three factors:

1. An immobilizing belief that government regulation is more effective than individual action
2. Lack of clear, credible guidance on powerful personal solutions
3. The problematic stigma that sustainable living is expensive, inconvenient, socially isolating, and an all-or-nothing pursuit requiring absolute perfection

All of these limiting beliefs create and propagate a dangerous and defeatist ethos of "why bother?" So instead of realizing the precious individual influence that got us into this planetary pickle in the first place, we sit back and literally watch the world burn, hoping that some big shot will step in, pick up the pieces, or, at the very least, pour us a stiff drink.

WHY YOU SHOULD
GIVE A SHIT

I had originally conceptualized this book to be about how to make eco-friendly living stylish and fun. Then, on the eve of November 8, 2016, whilst drowning my disbelief in endless glasses of raspberry vodka and soda along with millions of others around the globe, it became abundantly clear that the concept needed to shift because, holy crap, the stakes were raised exponentially in, like, four hours. Now, this isn't a political tome, but to cover sustainability while

HOT IN HERRE

We hear the term a ton, but let's take a closer look at what global warming actually means. Since pretty much the beginning of time, sunlight shone on the earth's surface has been radiated back into the atmosphere as heat. Naturally occurring levels of atmospheric gasses trap some of this heat while allowing the rest to escape into space. Global warming occurs when an overabundance of heat-trapping gasses like carbon dioxide and methane are present in the atmosphere. These greenhouse gasses (GHGs) are dubbed as such because they affect the transfer of infrared energy, letting in light while trapping heat, much like—you guessed it—a greenhouse. This exchange, or greenhouse effect, first discovered in the nineteenth century, is essential for keeping the earth habitable. Without it, the planet would be a brisk 60°F cooler.[i]

Climate change is related, but the terms (and occurrences) are not interchangeable. As planetary temperature climbs, winds and currents circulate heat in ways that can cool, warm, and alter the amount of rain and snowfall in different ways, resulting in changing climates depending upon the area. Climate change is best illustrated through ice caps rapidly melting in the Arctic while India simultaneously experiences unprecedented rainfall—two vastly different geographies experiencing significant changes to their localized climates as a result of global warming.

ignoring a US presidential administration that denies climate change or thwarts efforts to alleviate environmental burden would be to pen a fantasy fiction book. And that, this is not.

While the term *global warming* (accurately) alludes to a worldwide problem necessitating international action, much of the information in the following pages focuses on the United States. And no, this isn't because I'm touting some sort of ethnocentric agenda here; rather, this attention is because Americans are disproportionately responsible for climate change, very recently dethroning China for the infamous designation as the biggest carbon polluter in history. Accounting for only 4 percent of the world's 7.5 billion people, Americans create 14.34 percent of harmful global emissions.[2] We're like an uninvited, empty-handed party crasher who drinks the pricey craft beer and vomits all over the host's bed. Despite our size, the belief that four-car garages and nightly steak dinners are the apex of realizing the American dream has put us at the head of the class when it comes to fucking up the planet. And although this sounds grim, it's important to remember that the same behaviors that got us into this mess are the very things we need to harness to fix it. Because humans are impressionable community dwellers, heavily influenced by our peers, individual behaviors can quickly become collective movements. Just as tossing plastic bags and driving gas-guzzling cars are the current norms, we can cut the shit on an individual level and watch as our more sustainable behaviors go viral among the masses like an internet cat meme.

World on Fire

Global temperatures remained at manageable levels until the end of the last Ice Age some seven thousand years ago, which also ushered in human civilizations. Research overwhelmingly supports that human influence and emissions attendant with the rise of industrialism have significantly accelerated global warming. The burning of fossil fuels and carbon emissions have led to a 2°C temperature rise since the nineteenth century, most of which has happened in just the past thirty-five years, with sixteen of the seventeen warmest years on record occurring since 2001.[3] Given the planet's success in self-regulation over seven hundred thousand years and the intersection of people, industry, and rapid warming in a comparatively short period of time, it's pretty bananas to think that anyone capable of critical thinking is a climate change denier.

You might be thinking, *But hasn't the earth been warming for, like, forever?* Sure, the planet's been heating and cooling on its own for millions and millions of years, usually due to very small orbital variations that alter solar exposure. But these rhythmic shifts only averaged about 9°F and happened gradually over hundreds of thousands of years. What we're experiencing today is like going from putzing around on a golf cart to careening down the Autobahn in the Concorde.[4] And Mother Earth, like any woman scorned, has some pretty savage ways of showing us she's mad as hell and she's not gonna take it anymore:

Natural disasters: Hurricanes, tornadoes, drought, tsunamis, earthquakes, and flooding are all sorta part of the living-on-earth deal. However, climate change increases and intensifies the impact and frequency of these catastrophic events. For instance, serious droughts increase the likelihood of wildfires, and warming ocean currents can whip a category 3 storm into a city-shattering category 4. The frequency and severity of North American hurricanes alone has upped dramatically since the 1980s.[5]

Melting ice caps and glaciers: Greenland and Antarctic ice sheets have collectively decreased by some ninety cubic miles since 2002, and glaciers globally, from the Alps to the Himalayas, are literally withering away.[6] Yeah, those sad videos you see of disoriented polar bears roaming cracked ice? Not CGI, folks. This is real shit.

Dangerous seas: Atmospheric temps aren't the only things heating up. Oceans also absorb heat trapped in the atmosphere, and earth's seas have warmed an additional 0.302°F since 1969. And hey, news-flash, those ice caps and glaciers I just mentioned melt into water, so as the temperature and oceans warm, sea levels rise. Over the last two decades, sea levels have risen eight inches, a rate double that of the last century. Rising temps and harmful emissions have also led to a 30 percent increase in ocean acidity, which, I promise, will not make your next beach vacation very fun.[7]

Suffering habitats and species extinction: The earth is biodynamic and symbiotic. As climates dramatically shift, habitats shrink

SEA OF PLASTIC

It's been said that every piece of plastic ever produced (nine-plus billion tons since 1950, to be exact) still exists on the planet. As if that's not yikes-worthy enough, more than eight million tons of plastic are dumped into and added to our oceans every dang year. Discarded fishing supplies, litter, and even improperly recycled plastics make their way to the sea, where currents whip them into masses like the Great Pacific Garbage Patch, aka the Pacifica trash vortex, occupying an estimated 270,000 square miles (about the size of my home state of Texas) to more than 5,800,000 square miles (that's almost 8 percent of the Pacific Ocean, guys). Uncertainty about sizing is because most of the plastic particles are suspended at or just beneath the surface, making it difficult to detect by air craft or satellite. And that's just the near-surface plastic. What's going down on the ocean floor is largely unknown, but it's hypothesized to be a similar shit show. These pelagic plastics introduce harmful chemicals and threaten and kill wildlife, with an estimated five tons of plastic debris being

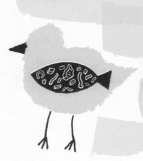

fed to albatross chicks on the Midway Atoll alone each year. These ocean plastics also facilitate the spread of invasive species who literally hitch a ride on pieces and float long distances to colonize other, foreign ecosystems. If we keep this shit up, the UN Ocean Conference estimated that by 2050 we could have more pieces of plastic than fish in the ocean. So if you're wondering why I continually recommend you avoid plastics at all cost, well, now you know why, homie.[ii]

(hence all of those sad polar bear photos you're seeing) or become inhospitable to indigenous species. As prey animals and life-sustaining plants die off, predators have two crummy choices: starve or roam in search of new terrain. Our planet's delicate ecosystem is a lot like Jenga: remove a few key pieces from the arrangement, and the structure becomes unstable; remove many, and it's not long before the whole thing comes crashing down. (In case metaphors aren't your thing, let me spell that out for you: plants, animals, and humans are all planetary Jenga pieces.) So it's really not all that dramatic to say that the end result of unmitigated climate change is bad-news bears for more than just bears.

Everyday experience also provides us with anecdotal evidence of global warming. As I write this, Chicago—a city renowned for its subzero winters (and its sausage-chomping football fans)—recently had its first snowless January and February in nearly 150 years.[8] If you're thinking that none of these phenomena are tied to human influence, that it's all a grand coincidence, I call bullshit. The very nature of life on earth is symbiotic.

Heightened risk of exploitation: Here's a goody to pull out during your next contentious Thanksgiving table conversation: climate change is an issue of global security. Severe droughts, famine, and natural disasters choke resources and can force mass migration, which leave people frantic for jobs, food, and security. And desperation makes people do crazy shit. How does this relate to global conflict? Imagine you're a Syrian wheat farmer. Life is pretty good until your rural area gets too hot or flooded to grow your crops. After trying, to no avail, to sell the saddest harvest ever, you pick up your family and migrate to a city where you attempt to get a different gig, despite having only specialized agrarian skills. Unsurprisingly, jobs are about as scarce as resources, and now you're really afraid that your family is going to starve, until one day a well-fed-looking guy with a machine gun tells you how ISIS gave him purpose and protection in exchange for his participation. You pick up what I'm putting down here? Climate change creates the fragility and instability necessary for militarized factions like ISIS and Boko Haram to recruit people and thrive.[9]

And because it just wouldn't be a party without administering some disproportionate blows to the poor, the impact of climate change, like so many things, will adversely impact those living in physically lower-lying, less developed, less economically prosperous areas. Wealthier countries, like the United States, utilize huge amounts of and profit from fossil fuels but don't do their fair share to address the detrimental effects of said usage, while poorer countries, especially those in low-lying areas more likely to be impacted by rising sea levels, who use little fossil fuels, will be the first to bear the worst impacts of climate change.[10]

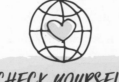

CHECK YOURSELF

If you're shaking your head and saying, "Not me, blondie," I encourage you to calculate your carbon footprint and see for yourself. Sites such as carbonfootprint.com take into account energy consumption, transportation use, shopping and dietary habits, and more to generate your, your household's, and even your business's carbon footprints. And the results are . . . eye opening. If your score is not-so-great right now, don't despair: giving a shit will help you turn the tide.

THE SOLUTION IS YOU

If there's anything I want to leave you with after you read this book, it's the belief that your actions are powerful. As evidenced by everything I've laid out above, human emissions and greed have royally screwed the planet. Surely, then, humans making sustainable shifts can unfuck the world. And by doing so, you'll also help habitats, animals, and people. And if you're the kind of person who needs further "What's in it for me?" incentive before you buy into this whole "giving a shit" thing, I've got that for you, too. Living more minimally, with attention to environmental impact, benefits you in many, many rad ways. My first year of going balls-out and employing the strategies herein, I saved almost $15,000. Bidding adieu to my car, shopping from local markets and bulk bins, buying mostly secondhand, and minimizing my purchases wasn't difficult—in fact, it was liberating and happened to leave a lot more green in my pocket. And for those of you wondering, no, that is not enough savings to buy your own personal helicopter. But it makes sense: buying fewer and better often means buying less, saving you money and, arguably, more precious time. Moreover, I felt less stressed (because I wasn't as saddled and stymied by rampant, senseless consumption), healthier (because I replaced my love for fast-food animal products with more of the whole, real, from-the-ground goodness), and more aligned with my values than ever, which had and continues to have serious "my life has meaning!" moments.

How to Give a Shit

When I first embarked on this exploration, I found some cool books that showed me how to not make trash or create my own cruelty-free cosmetics. But there wasn't anything that holistically combined niche elements from different schools of sustainable thought to create an accessible road map to a healthier, streamlined, stress-free, and sustainable existence. Basically, *Give a Sh*t* is the kind of book I wanted when I was exploring how to be the best version of myself, and it will hopefully be your buddy through your transition to a kinder, more conscious life.

Some of the terms I use throughout the book may be ones you've heard of before, and others may be new to you. Together, these ideologies form the Give a Shit philosophy and aim to be your North Star as you gently, gradually shift your behaviors to support lasting change:

Animal friendly: Whether it's adopting a more plant-based, vegetarian, or vegan diet; eschewing animal materials and ingredients in goods; buying only cruelty-free personal care and home products; adopting an animal at your local shelter; or all of the above, Give a Shit gives you practical advice on how to be a better protector of our animal friends through every aspect of your life. So if you find that animals start nuzzling you at parties and following you home, you know who to thank (me).

Minimalist: Living better with less. It's a mantra that's gained momentum in our ever-chaotic world of pushed consumption. From decluttering your space (and maybe your mind, as a result), to buying and owning fewer items (but of better quality), to considering population burden, a cornerstone of giving a shit is paring down to the essentials to allow for the clarity necessary to make solid, values-based purchasing and life decisions. From the items you own to the company you keep, when you only allow things that truly matter to make their way into your life, you save precious time and energy. If this philosophy hadn't become my way of life, there's no way I could've written this book while maintaining a full-time job and not totally pissing off my dog, friends, and family.

Low and zero waste: From repurposing, buying secondhand, reusing, recycling, composting, eschewing disposables, donating, collaborative consumption, and supporting closed-loop circular manufacturing, living a less wasteful life is a main tenet of the Give a Shit lifestyle. Suggestions in this book will guide you toward significantly reducing the waste you put into the world and landfills. In other words, we're all gonna get a lot less trashy. Bless up.

People forward: Whether you're purchasing a diamond ring, bed frame, or a carton of strawberries, this book gives you the necessary knowledge to make decisions that support fair wages, safe working conditions, healthy communities, upward mobility, and anti-slavery and exploitation initiatives for people at home and abroad. Moreover, philanthropy is a cornerstone of not only a life well lived but of the Give a Shit mantra. From donating items to people who can truly use them, to supporting and engaging in social justice activism, to adopting healthier habits that promote wellness and reduced stress, this book is full of strategies that move equality and fairness forward in electrifying ways.

Location considerate: Whether you're opting for Made in the USA, eating like a locavore, supporting smaller businesses and makers, or traveling the globe lightly, Give a Shit considers where things are made or harvested, the lengths they (and we) travel, eco-friendly transportation options, and the jobs those choices create and sustain.

Eco-friendly: From choosing innovative materials and goods made from postconsumer content, to making simple dietary shifts that significantly reduce climate-warming emissions, to using personal care products that assimilate safely into waterways and soil, you can make more environmentally sound choices with the tools and knowledge in this handy guide.

And I give it to you straight. Guidance for a comfortable eco-home, polished ethical wardrobe, and cruelty-free grooming routine, easily digestible advice to have a professional persona and social life aligned with purpose, and only the recipes you need to blow people's minds for all of life's occasions. Full of helpful tips, entertaining anecdotes, and plenty of swearing, this book is like getting juicy advice from your cool, slightly skanky friend (me) over a lovely ~~glass~~ bottle of wine—delivered with plenty of gusto but sans any bullshit judgment, ultimatums, or wacky expectations of perfection.

You see, I'm not going to tell you that in order to make a difference you need to go all or nothing—because that's just untrue. This isn't a diet book or a corporate HR manual. Sure, I'll help you get your sustainable shit together, but here's a list of things I won't do:

→ Slap you on the wrist or take you on an in-law-style guilt trip for stuff you've done in the past—today we start fresh

→ Your laundry or taxes

→ Instruct you to eschew cool things like booze, wild shindigs, mind-expanding travel, beautiful clothes, mouthwatering food, or luxurious digs

In fact, being the life lover that I am, I'm going to encourage you to engage, imbibe, and go to town on all the things that make life a radical journey. This isn't a manual of restrictions—it's a manifesto for a life that's, perhaps for the first time, in harmony with your desire to do good.

JUDGE THE COVER

This physical book is a faithful embodiment of what's inside: it's printed on 100 percent recycled, FSC-certified paper and with nontoxic vegetable-based inks. It was also printed in North America at a hydropowered printing facility. This baby walks the walk! It's also light and compact enough to carry with you when you need an on-the-go hit of inspiration, pretty and accessible enough for gifting (or just passing along to a friend when you're finished with it), and thick and coaster-y enough to use as a, well, coaster in a pinch. Just please don't throw it in the trash. That would be the ultimate irony, and unlike that Alanis Morrissette song, I hate that shit.

Who Am I to Tell You to Give a Shit?

You know those tabloids that are, like, "Celebrities! They're just like us!" that show a supermodel with a small, singular cellulite dimple or Rod Stewart using a public restroom, and somehow we're supposed to feel better or like we have a sudden kinship with them? Well, I'm no celebrity, and I do have some cellulite and have used a public restroom before, but here's the part where I tell you of my decidedly un-eco-beginnings in an effort to show you that if I can do it, hot damn, anyone can.

I wasn't born with a clear-eyed view on sustainability. Hell, I didn't even know what the word meant until I entered my late teens. I grew up in Texas, where everyone is basically breastfed beef. That said, my mother was an animal lover through and through who brought home strays like it was her job (it wasn't). At one point I shared my childhood home with a collection of sassy stray cats (like, deadly, bite-your-finger-off sassy), a one-eyed dachshund named Ginger, a gun-shy German shorthaired pointer named Susie with a crooked toe, a half-bobcat named Thomas, two hermit crabs, two box turtles, and one very unhappy catfish. It was an ever-so-slightly unconventional environment that instilled my love for animals early on. We'd always adopted companion animals, but I hadn't made the connection between the pets with whom I shared bedtime stories and walks around the neighborhood (not the catfish) and the creatures on my plate. Like a good southerner, I was pretty meat-and-dairy focused in my eating habits (fave meal: Hamburger Helper Beef Stroganoff with a tall glass of whole milk) and never gave that a second thought. I even had my high school graduation dinner at Fogo de Chão, one of those places where waiters dressed as gauchos present you with a meat feast of Versailles-esque proportions, where I proceeded to shove as many of God's creatures into my mouth as humanly possible. Date me.

But underneath my rampant carnivorous streak, I was an animal lover, protector, and defender—a level-10 vegan just waiting to happen. My first gateway drug into giving a shit happened when I was eleven years old, excitedly meandering the snack cake aisle (yes, an entire aisle) of my local grocery store. There, stuck to the floor with muddy boot prints, was a flier outlining the gory reality of animal testing. Clearly discarded by someone who didn't want to be bothered, I peeled the pamphlet off the floor and, intrigued, had my first introduction to the seedy and cruel world of animal exploitation. I couldn't believe that rabbits, mice, dogs, and cats, among others, were all experimented on to the point of injury and death for cosmetic and pharmaceutical efficacy.

So there I was—I had the information, I knew that the practice felt wrong to me, and from that point on, I never knowingly used another animal-tested product. This was in the nineties, and the cruelty-free movement wasn't as prominent as it is today, so I spent much of my only-child youth talking to my dogs, listening to seventies AM favorites on a little pink radio (which makes me a formidable karaoke partner), and making my own lotions and other beauty concoctions. You know, like any normal kid. This odd education seeded an early desire to learn how to make everything from home cleaners to lipstick better, safer, and with more eco-panache. My first foray into green business was when my friend Jenny and I made homemade cruelty-free lip balms and sold them to our classmates for a cool $5 a pop. I wasn't popular AT ALL, but that week, when even the mean girls took a break from making fun of my stringy bangs and flat chest to clamor for our creations, I felt, for a split second, like I had arrived. Mind you, this was just a stepping stone. I was still eating meat with abandon and wearing my patchwork leather "cool kid" jacket (that really made me look like a middle-aged 1970s taxi driver, but I digress) to school. I was taking baby steps, which is why this book never takes a dickhead all-or-nothing approach: you take the steps you are ready to take, and you keep going.

This journey continued and expanded into adulthood. By all

accounts I'd done all the right things—paid bills on time, not housed a meth lab, created a cool career as a political strategist, and basically was a pretty contributive member of society (vodka-fueled 3 a.m. Air Supply karaoke solos in the street aside). But a huge part of me wanted more, and as I began to explore how fun, easy, and impactful environmentally friendly living can be, I found my purpose.

I spent much of my twenties traveling for work whilst carving out time to learn how other cultures adapt to, beautify, and respect their environments. I studied indigenous beauty and culinary rituals, got loads of mosquito bites, and made out with guys who had cool accents and overwhelming colognes. The biggest takeaway from these adventures, however, was how the rest of the world seems to have us beat with the whole "living better with less" thing. In Western societies we see *everything* as disposable—from our morning coffee cup to our clothes to our mattresses (and to get really deep, even our relationships)—and it's literally killing the planet and our overall happiness. New studies emerge every day tackling how we are depleting the ozone, contributing to the exploitation of animals and workers, and becoming increasingly more depressed because we value stuff, comparison, and status over contentment, charity, and gratitude. It sounds heavy because it is.

And that's why I'm here writing this book. Not just because I believe that everyone is capable of making small shifts that can encourage powerful change but also because much of the eco-guidance out there can be so darned preachy, crunchy as hell in a way that scares people (even me), straight-up judgmental, or simply not relatable (not all of us have ten hours to mill our own flour). After rocking communications for politicians for years, I've developed a different approach—one that's warm, fun, and understanding while still being well researched. I got a master's in evidence-based social intervention to learn how to employ data to understand whether little behavioral changes on a person-to-person scale actually yield greater impact (verdict: they do). I got another degree in holistic health so I could speak more fluently on foods that are not only nourishing but also support (rather than fuck up) our ecosystem. And I've honed my own lifestyle strategies over the past twenty years to develop a sustainable, compassionate wardrobe, grooming regimen, comfortable and aesthetically pleasing home, and recipe repertoire that completely knock my (and others') socks off. Because the blog life was a bit too navel gazing, "preaching to the choir" for me, I took my message to mainstream outlets and have done hundreds of television segments over the past three years focused on showing people how simple and fun giving a shit can be. I'm not trying to toot my own horn like I'm some know-it-all, eco–David Koresh here, either. I'm simply stating the facts, ma'am: I know this shit. I live this shit. I've been bringing this shit to the masses in a fun and friendly way that actually gets results. Why? Because I genuinely believe in the power of us and the urgency of now.

Who Should Give a Shit?

You. Your family. Your pals. Your frenemies. Your climate change–denying cousin who thinks recycling is something created by the Devil to put plastic companies out of business. Your grandmother, who, if she's anything like my 107-year-old Nonna, still washes and reuses tinfoil (the eco-OG, if ever there was one). Your coworkers who won't stop using fifteen Styrofoam cups a day despite you buying them reusable water bottles. That Bumble date you never called again because he threw a Gatorade bottle off the train platform in an effort to "impress you."

Because we've got a big job to do, there's plenty of room for everyone—no matter how rich, busy, or connected—to give a shit. And it's something everyone can fit into their lifestyle. For instance, if you get to the kitchen chapter and you're like, "Nope, too hard," I urge you to explore other areas of your life in which you can make some simple swaps. And if you're the type who wants immediate gratification with low investment, each chapter ends with Quick Hits, impactful changes that take less than five minutes.

YOUR LITTLE GREEN BOOK

Throughout the book, I make mention of a mysterious, alluring Little Black Book. Even better than a collection of hotties' numbers, this one is full of my favorite Give a Sh*t-worthy products, brands, stores, and resources. Since that list is always growing and evolving, I've housed it on the interwebs so it'll stay fresh (and relevant) AF for years to come. Access it at www.ashleepiper.com/LBB.

WE ARE THE ONES
WE HAVE BEEN WAITING FOR

As I attended the Women's March in Washington, DC, on January 21, 2017, I held a banner emblazoned with one of my favorite Alice Walker quotes: *We are the ones we have been waiting for.* And it hit me: while we've been conditioned to wait for our elected officials to legislate solutions for us, we can take action—powerful, positive, unstoppable action—right freaking now, regardless of who's in

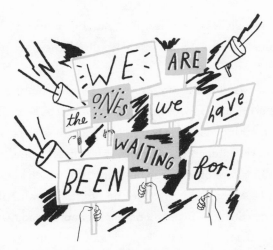

office or holding the purse strings. The truth remains that no one can stop us from adopting sustainable personal habits that ignite to have a collective influence. And the more we develop this individual accountability, not only will we realize that the embers of lasting change burn brightly within us, but we'll also have the courage, confidence, and community to continually seek out innovative solutions to complex ecological issues. If you're nodding your head, you're already with me. And there are millions of people just like us who need only a little nudge to flint the sparks within. We're solutionaries, and we're not content to let apathy and inaction discourage us from doing what's right and what's so desperately needed.

So it's time to get real. This is the moment to face down the doomsday climate change Leviathan with pluck and passion. We're going to get through this together, and we're going to feel great, have near-criminal amounts of fun, save some coin, and look boss while saving the planet. Take my hand, shit-giver, and let's go. We've been waiting for you.

Give a Shit:

In Your Home

Your home should be a sanctuary, a space emblematic of your style that inspires ideas, relaxation, and connection. A place where you can entertain and retreat, whip up fancy meals and enjoy hangover pizza, raise kiddos or a pot of basil, and everything in between. Sure, that sounds good, especially the pizza part. "But Ashlee, what if my home is an unfinished basement with leaky faucets that comes with a close-talker landlord, and I'm broke as a joke?" Dude, that sounds like my first apartment (did said landlord steal your bras from the laundry room too?). I promise we can still turn your space into an eco-efficient and inspiring haven without a lot of cash or hassle. Think of your abode as your own eco-laboratory. This is where you'll experiment with and fine-tune the strategies that work for you—at your own pace, with your people, before you bring them out into the wild.

In an ideal world I could come to your house sporting a bushel of aromatherapeutic cleaners and a killer Spotify playlist and personally whip your space into Give a Shit shape (something from which I would derive ridiculous amounts of pleasure). But alas,

THE AVERAGE AMERICAN HOUSEHOLD

Considering that the United States comprises only 4.5 percent of the world's population, it may strike you (hopefully) as crazy egregious that we use 18 percent of the world's energy and produce 14.34 percent of harmful global emissions.[i] To shed some light on why making sustainable shifts at home matters, let's check out some stats related to resource consumption and waste habits in the average American home. Our little US households use 38 percent of the country's energy. When indirect usage is accounted for, like energy used elsewhere to produce food or move water to homes, that number jumps to 80 percent of total country-wide energy consumption.[ii] So, ya know, our households are a good place to reign in our consumption habits. On average a typical household in the United States:

❋ *Uses 11,700 kWh of power each year. That's double what French households and triple what Chinese households consume. It's especially egregious when you consider that 1.1 billion people worldwide don't even have access to electricity.[iii]*

❋ *Tosses 25 percent, or $2,275, of uneaten groceries every year. Every single day Americans waste enough food to fill the Rose Bowl (that's a ninety-thousand-seat football stadium, for the less sport-inclined among us).[iv]*

❋ *Doesn't compost to the tune of 72 percent, but cite a willingness to do so if composting were easier (hint: it is! Keep reading. I dish the dirt on composting on page 36).[v]*

❋ *Occupies a median twenty-five-hundred-square-foot home containing an average of three hundred thousand items. And because of all that stuff, 9 percent of households utilize or rent external storage space.[vi]*

❋ *Has 1.8 cars, 98 percent of which guzzle gas, as opposed to being hybrid or electric.[vii]*

that's probably not gonna happen. Luckily, though, you have this book, which is the next best thing.

In this chapter we'll touch on the habits and swaps that make any home more sustainable without costing a ton of money or time. These tips and tricks combine an optimal blend of minimalism, organization, and sustainability. From acing composting and recycling, to finally understanding and winning at energy efficiency, to paring down and furnishing your place with a new philosophical rubric, you'll be armed with information that applies to and revitalizes any space, whether you own a mansion or rent an RV. Approach this as a Choose Your Own Adventure book—pick the strategies and tips that seem doable and applicable within your lifestyle (or, better yet, the lifestyle you've always wanted), and build from there. Not every one of these suggestions will work for everyone. Sometimes you rent and it's impossible to control the amount of insulation in your space, no matter how many passive aggressive texts you send your landlord. Other times you're simply not in the market for new windows or a factory-fresh fridge. But don't let these challenges discourage you. There are plenty of juicy, cheap, totally easy tips for everyone, no matter your living arrangement, so I encourage you to get creative. (Also, save this book for when you win the lottery or sign that big record deal and are in a position to make those choices and purchases.) Okay, now I feel like the hype man in a late-eighties infomercial, but seriously, this chapter is the springboard for your leaner, greener, shit-giving life.

RECYCLING AND COMPOSTING

Strategizing an eco-forward life and home begins with thinking about the end of things. No, not in the same way you did when you went through your high school Robert Smith–idolizing goth phase.

It means thinking about where your refuse goes and how it makes its way there through your actions. Look at your trash can for a hot minute. Go ahead, I'll wait. What do you see a lot of? In my non-eco-heyday, my waste culprits were (1) food and beverage packaging, (2) leftover food, and (3) non–food product packaging. From that simple scan I knew that the way forward was to (1) lessen my reliance on packaged goods, (2) find a solution for managing food scraps, and (3) ensure that any packaged items I did buy were at least reusable or recyclable. Pretty simple, right? When paired with simple behavioral shifts toward buying fewer packaged and unnecessary things, establishing manageable recycling and composting systems in your home will help you significantly reduce what you send to the landfill.

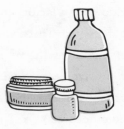

Recycling

If ever there was a phrase that I wish was banned from the English language, along with "That's what SHE said," it'd be "But I recycle!" Cool story, bro, but recycling alone will not save the planet. The truth is that the actual impact of recycling is a lullaby, something that makes us feel good, but it isn't nearly as effective as we're led to believe, mostly because, as American humans, we're simply not that good at doing it correctly. Don't believe me? Peep the trash can at your nearest chain coffee shop. Although there are clearly marked, conveniently located recycle bins nearby, trash cans (often labeled "landfill" to really hit home to people where their toss leads) are usually overflowing with more misplaced plastic than a reality TV star's face. Sure, *some* of the 4.1 pounds of trash individual Americans produce every day can be recycled, but according to the US Environmental Protection Agency (EPA), even though 75 percent of our waste is recyclable, only 30 percent actually makes it into the recycling stream, and recycling requires a tremendous amount of energy. We treat recycling as a magic cure-all as opposed to the last resort it's intended to be.[1]

Now, I'm not saying that you shouldn't recycle or that you'll reach some grand master eco-status where you'll never have anything to dispose of. Even the most eco-expert among us will still have some items to recycle, and that's cool. But the important thing is to first reduce the amount of recyclables you purchase. Before we recycle, we need to think about refusing, reducing, and repurposing items already in our possession (and I cover that more in the coming sections). That said, please, please recycle absolutely anything you need to after you've exhausted the aforementioned three Rs. Here's the good news, folks: 94 percent of Americans have access to recycling services, 73 percent of which are curbside![2] How easy is that? In this day and age, there's really no excuse to not be recycling on the regular with precision and passion. It should be as innate as breathing or kissing—something we inherently know is an important part of our existence. And like breathing or kissing, the keys to success are doing it with precision and enthusiasm, which leads me to my next point.

WISHCYCLING

Contrary to popular belief, a recycle bin is not a wishing well or a lucky Italian fountain in which you toss coins, and your local recycling facility workers are not wizards who magically transform something completely unrecyclable into something that is. Sure, what recycling facilities can do is pretty freaking incredible, but putting any old item in the recyclables bin does not make it so. This practice is called wishcycling, and although I totally encourage you to keep wishin' and hopin' in other aspects of your glorious life, recycling simply doesn't work that way. Here's how recycling actually works:

Study up on what's recycled in your system: Most areas will recycle aluminum (beverage cans, cleaned foil, and aluminum cookware), steel and tin cans, corrugated cardboard, magazines, newspapers, office papers, paperboard, paper cardboard beverage cartons, envelopes sans plastic windows (so remove those before tossing the paper in the bin), phonebooks, glass (clear, amber, and emerald), and certain plastics (especially bottles, jars, and jugs). Some municipalities will recycle yard clippings, energy-efficient light bulbs, batteries, and electronics, but check before you put these out, especially as they might have separate pick-up days or requirements.

Know what separation your system demands: My city has single-stream recycling, so I can put my plastics, glass, metal, and paper in the same bin. That's not always the case, so get the 411 by calling 311.

Get the schedule: Knowing pick-up frequency ensures that your bins aren't overflowing, which can sometimes lead people to toss recyclables in the trash simply to cut down on clutter.

NOT REALLY RECYCLABLE

According to a Pew Research Center survey, 59 percent of Americans believe that "most types of items" can be recycled in their community.[viii] While there are some exceptions, here are some items that most areas will not recycle:

❋ **Styrofoam:** Also known as foamed polystyrene or plastic #6, Styrofoam can sit in a landfill for centuries. A few programs exist that can handle recycling this material, but they're not the norm. The best course of action? Avoid using Styrofoam and foam-coated items like packing peanuts, food containers, and coated cups.

❋ **Plastic caps:** Although your plastic bottle may be recyclable in your area, the cap is often made from very different plastic.

❋ **Plastic hangers:** These are usually a blend of plastics, so they're notoriously difficult to recycle. Repurpose or mend whenever possible.

❋ **Mirrors:** Mirrors aren't just glass, homie. They're full of reflective chemicals, so they cannot enter the traditional glass recycling stream.

❋ **Pyrex and ceramic:** These are types of glass that have been treated with chemicals to withstand high heat and, thus, cannot mix with traditional glass recycling.

❋ **Food-contaminated containers:** Alas, the grease from last night's pizza and pasta render your paper takeout containers and food boxes unrecyclable. Many composting programs and methods can handle these greasy bits if the paper itself is not mixed with inorganic material.

❋ **Shower curtains and liners:** Most of these are made from polyvinyl chloride (PVC), the world's most widely produced synthetic plastic polymer, which cannot be broken down again. So it's here forever as your moldy shower curtain. Cool. (I use a reusable, washable cloth shower liner to avoid this PVC-induced guilt; check out page 72 if you are intrigued.)

❋ **Photo paper:** Some mixed-recycling programs can handle newer photo paper, but traditional photo development uses chemicals that can't enter the recycling stream.

❋ **Incandescent light bulbs:** These bad boys are metal and glass in one and often contain mercury or lead.

❋ **Plastic and zip-top bags:** Most of these shopping and storage bags can be recycled, but they require a different system than that of most municipalities. Whenever possible, recycle these at specific drop-offs sometimes found at grocery stores and other retailers.

❋ **Tires:** When melted, tires emit toxic gasses, so they're not often accepted in municipal recycling. Most tire suppliers will offer recycling options (or will just include it in your bill automatically) when you get them changed.

Check and disassemble: Know the recycling numbers on materials that are accepted in your community and adhere to them. And think of the components of packaging. For instance, a bottle may be plastic #1, while the cap or lid may be #6, which may not be recyclable in your area.

Get plastic savvy: It's a bummer, but the number on the bottom of plastics can't always be trusted. A good rule of thumb is to look at the shape of the container. Generally plastic bottles, jars, and jugs are recyclable.

Clean everything: Just like the sign in your office kitchen says, municipal waste workers are not your mom, and no, they're not interested in that last bit of salsa in the jar, so wash applicable recyclables before you put them in the bin. This also keeps your home from smelling like a literal Dumpster.

Be courteous: Real people often sort through our recyclables. Sharp objects like broken glass shards and razor blades can make someone's day horrible and scary, so don't be a dick: find another way to properly recycle those, like taking them to a specific drop-off for scrap glass or metal.

Seek out alternatives: For the items that your community recycling system doesn't support, explore other options. This may mean you stockpile certain recyclables (such as corks, certain plastics, and other items your municipality doesn't collect curbside) and take or mail them to a designated facility. Most hazardous materials, like batteries, paint, and motor oil, have special disposal requirements you can look up online. Harder-to-off-load items, like mattresses, don't need to be put out with the trash—peep my Ethical Off-load chart at ashleepiper.com/ethicaloffload for solid guidance on how to responsibly and consciously off-load anything.

Organize your home-based recycling center by end point: You'll need designated bins for your municipal recycling needs and also smaller repositories for items that get recycled or donated elsewhere. I keep small jars for collecting corks (which I donate to the animal shelter), batteries (which I recycle at a receptacle at my office), and those pesky silica packets (which I keep in case I drop my phone in water or need to dry out and defunk sweaty running shoes). Having these repositories all in one place doesn't have to be unsightly or complicated, and it ensures you are ready to recycle like a pro.

Don't forget the other rooms of the house: You only need one recycling area in your home, but don't forget to recycle nonkitchen items. Toiletry packaging, office papers and mail, toilet paper rolls, and other items can be easily recycled and sometimes composted.

RESEARCH ROTTING

Take five and research the compost options in your area. Folks with yards may be able to enjoy outdoor composting, while urban dwellers may have access to municipally supported composting (they bring you a bin along with trash and recycling receptacles), farmers' markets that will take your scraps (just keep them in the freezer and bring 'em over on market day), or subscription services (like mine, where a cool person on a bike picks up my compost bucket every two weeks). And then marvel at (1) how much more conscious you become about using up your food, and (2) how you'll become Sudoku-level obsessed with composting as many things as possible (including eccentric shit like drain-clogging hair, fingernails, and pencil shavings). Yep, things are about to get really fun up in here.

Composting

We are fortunate to live in a country of relative abundance. We're so abundant in food, in fact, that Americans throw away 40 percent of our food supply each year (that's an estimated 1,160 pounds of food per person every 365 days)—a sobering reality when you consider that one in six Americans (42 million total, including 13 million children and 5.4 million seniors) don't know from where they're getting their next meal and that many countries experience severe drought-induced famine or widespread hunger on the regular.[3] According to the Environmental Protection Agency (EPA), food waste is the single-biggest occupant of our country's landfills and a big source of methane emissions, a potent greenhouse gas that significantly contributes to climate change.[4] But help is on its way.

Riding in on its emerald steed is composting—an effective way to divert organic materials from the landfill, save energy, and help a local farmer (or garden, even if it's the potted plant on your windowsill). Composting also cuts down on the resources associated with transporting organic material to a landfill. In my area there's no longer a nearby landfill, so all of the city's trash is trucked out to a neighboring suburb, and that journey requires gas and oil, creates emissions, and costs taxpayers money.[5] In an effort to reduce this insanity, many areas have also begun charging residents for the amount of trash they create and number of trash cans they fill.[6] Although the charge may be negligible to some, composting will effectively cut your trash in half, if not more, and it saves precious resources. And with so many options, from sleek outdoor composters, to discreet, non-smelly in-home receptacles, to farmers' markets that will gladly take your scraps year-round, composting is cleaner, cooler, and less stinky than ever before.

TAKE A KNEE

Now that your recycling and composting systems are good to go, it's time to spread the knowledge far and wide, like to your housemates. Wrangle your peeps and have a quick, Boy Scout–style huddle whereby you walk through the system and lay out the dos and don'ts. This not only ensures that everyone is on the same page (no cigarette butts in the compost, Grandpa Mickey) but also is a great opportunity to teach little ones (and not so little ones) about their important role in protecting the planet. So take a knee, ply people with cookies, and prepare yourself for smooth sailing.

ENERGY EFFICIENCY

Modern technology definitely deserves a high five. Such advances keep our indoor climates cozy, help us whip up dope smoothies and avocado toast, and enable *Game of Thrones* binge-watching sessions and funny dog-video sharing with the touch of a button. But, if we're honest, we've perhaps become a little too reliant on our technological treasures. Americans (as in, *each* of us) use 4,500 kWh of power in our homes every year. That's almost triple the usage of our German and UK counterparts and eight and a half times the usage of peeps in Brazil, Mexico, and China.[7] Magical as powered-up devices and appliances are, it's time we consider and cull our disproportionate consumption. Here are some easy ways to cut down on the resource- and cost-leeching behaviors and devices that contribute to unnecessary environmental burden, all without making your life completely cumbersome or unfun.

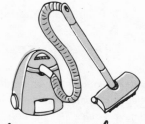

Appliances and Devices

→ **Explore energy alternatives**: Say you are addicted to coffee (points to self). Does said coffee taste better when it's made in one of those wasteful K-Cup things or via a no-energy-required French press? Answer: no. Explore your personal rituals and see if there are low- or no-energy alternatives that require little sacrifice but are way kinder to the planet and your wallet.

→ **Have only what you regularly use**: Despite my best intentions, I am not, in fact, making crêpes or dehydrating fruit every week. I also don't really print or microwave anything; thus, I don't need a crêpe maker, electric food dehydrator, laser printer, or a microwave. Your needs will likely be different, so realistically assess what you actually use on the regular. Donate or sell everything you don't need.

→ **Unplug**: Did you know that an estimated 8 percent (and $100) of your annual electricity bill is due to items not in use that are plugged in? Avoid this energy suck (called peripheral or phantom energy drain) by unplugging items you're not using. For those items to which you need instant access, like computers, televisions, and sound systems, use an eco-power strip, which allows you to disconnect peripheral items from the power source completely with the touch of a button, thereby saving you dough and reducing carbon consumption.[8]

→ **Rethink cable:** I'm sure I'll have a bunch of pitchforks and torches outside my house for this one, but the average cable box/DVR combo uses about 446 kWh a year, which is more than the average refrigerator (around 415 kWh/year) and second only to air-conditioning units (1,500-plus kWh/year) in terms of highest power use in the typical household. I'm not saying you need to or should give up TV completely; I'm saying stay mindful and remember that instant use means "always on," which requires a ton of energy.[9] Perhaps some of the handy-dandy subscription streaming services will be enough tube for you to say farewell to the cable box forever? Consider it food for thought.

→ **Try repairs first:** TVs, phones, computers, and tablets are dope as hell, but is it really necessary that we have the newest versions the minute they debut? Most of the time what we have works well, and buying brand new creates production and disposal burden. If the newest thing will save you time, is essential for your job, or is deeply important to you, then go for it. If it's not, often a system update or upgrade to your existing devices will give you the functionality and speed you need.

→ **Rethink traditional usage:** Your fridge isn't a late-night club. Get in, get out, and keep the door shut as much as possible to minimize the 7 percent energy use (about 50 to 120 kWh per year, if you're into energy terms) caused by the compressor having to drive out warm air. To put that waste into perspective, 50 kWh of energy could run your dishwasher twenty times and your washing machine twenty-five times (that's basically a free load of laundry every other week for an entire year).[10]

→ **Skip the preheat:** Unless you're a professional baker, it's not necessary to preheat your oven every single time you bake or roast. Save that natural gas, electricity, and cash for more finicky or yeast-based recipes that require a preheated oven.

→ **Keep your appliances in good repair:** Clean the coils on your fridge and ensure there's enough clearance for ventilation, replace filters in your climate system and vacuums, and clear the crumbs from your toaster. A little bit of maintenance prevents grime and debris from clogging and making your devices work harder than they need to, which—you guessed it—requires a lot more energy.

→ **Buy secondhand:** If you've ever tried to dispose of an old dishwasher or oven, you know how difficult it can be to close the loop on large appliances. So whenever possible, opt for refurbished or secondhand versions.

→ **Invest in energy-efficient:** Sometimes buying new is the only logical aesthetic and investment option. Opt for Energy Star appliances with solid warranty and repair options (and look into tax breaks and rebates for such purchases). Be sure to select the appropriate size and capacity for your space, and read the Energy Guide label to compare the energy consumption of competing models.

→ **Consider resource sharing:** Borrowing is cool again, and it's an excellent way to lessen clutter in your home and environmental resource drain. Items you don't use every day but might occasionally want, like a bread maker or juicer, could be your neighbors' daily staples (and vice versa). Some communities have "stuff libraries," where folks can check out items like power tools; landscaping, sports, and crafting equipment; and other items that are nice to have occasionally but that you don't need every day. This sort of program strengthens community bonds (which, let's be real, we can all use more of) and ensures your streamlined home stays that way. No stuff library in your 'hood? I feel your pain. Start your own, or just knock on your neighbor's door before going out to buy a big-ticket item like a snow blower or food dehydrator.

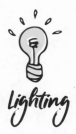

Lighting

If the rise of insta-starlets and reality television stars has taught us anything, it's that good lighting can work miracles. Although you're probably not looking to stage your home for the perfect selfie, eco-friendly lighting swaps will not only beautify your space but also save you beaucoup bucks. It's estimated that 10 percent of the energy we consume residentially is for lighting.[11]

→ **Cut 'em**: Your dad was right: he does not, in fact, own the power company. So although it sounds damn simple, turning lights off when not in use is an excellent way to—you guessed it—conserve resources and save money. If you're impossibly forgetful, explore smart bulb systems, which allow you to alter brightness and usage from your mobile devices when you're away from home.

→ **Dim it**: If you're in a space where you can change up the wiring, opting for dimmer switches wherever possible can save you about $40 per year[12] and might just help you get laid more often.

→ **Bulb better**: Swap traditional incandescent bulbs, which only burn for about a thousand hours, for energy-efficient, longer-lasting versions. And if cost is a worrying factor for renters, remember that you can unscrew them and take them with you when you move.

- Halogen incandescent: Great for spaces in which lights are turned on and off frequently (e.g., hallways and bathrooms), their light is similar to that of traditional incandescents, but halogens use about 28 percent less energy and last between one to three years.
- Energy Star–rated compact fluorescent bulbs (CFLs): Those swirly, soft-serve ice cream cone–looking bulbs use 75

percent less energy, burn for ten thousand hours, have a lifespan of seven to eleven years, and an overall savings of $53 per bulb. But they do contain mercury and can be hazardous when broken, FYI.

- Light-emitting diodes (LEDs): More expensive (like $30 a bulb) but also the most energy-efficient choice, boasting up to fifty thousand hours of use, a twenty-three-year lifespan, and an overall savings of $137 per bulb.[13] Damn, Gina.

→ **Go solar**: Explore solar options, which harness sunlight to power fixtures. Sun-powered and recharging residential options are popping up everywhere, from panels you can mount on your roof to simple outdoor lighting that means you'll never be fumbling for your keys in the dark outside your front door again.

→ **Be natural**: Photographers love it for a reason. Whenever possible, bring in and exploit natural light. Sheer curtains, skylights, and mirrors make the most of sunshine and can even make your space appear larger.

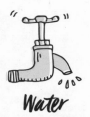

Water

H_2O is sort of essential to life, and many of us are hella fortunate to live in areas where potable water is available in abundant supply. Such abundance can lead us to think that water is a commodity in endless supply, but if you've read this far, you know that's definitely not true. Whether you're worried about keeping your bill low or conserving a vital and precious planetary resource, here are some ways you can keep the metaphorical glass half full:

→ **Tap that**: Use the magical tap water we're so lucky to have. If your local water quality isn't so hot, loads of rad water filtration options exist, from charcoal sticks to pitchers that filter 240 gallons of water a year for about 19 cents a day.[14]

→ **Disable your fridge's ice maker and water dispenser**: A simple ice tray makes arguably better cubes *and* saves water and energy. And let's be real: those freezer-made ice cubes can start to taste and smell pretty funky after a while, which is a real party foul.

→ **Ensure your plumbing is in good shape**: Drips can be an annoying drag (and can haunt your dreams). If you have a hunch your plumbing is inefficient, here are some quick diagnostics:

- If you have access to your water meter, do an initial reading and follow up two hours later when you haven't used any water. If the meter reading has changed, you've got a leak.
- To check for a toilet leak, put food coloring into the tank. If color appears in the bowl without flushing, you've got a leak (and a disturbingly red toilet now).
- If you have leaks you're not able to repair immediately, catch the water in a bucket and use it to water plants or flush the toilet.

→ **Install low-flow shower heads**: Showering accounts for nearly 17 percent of residential water use, and conventional shower heads flow at five-plus gallons per minute. An affordable, low-flow option still gives you a good dousing and can save anywhere from one-half to two and a half gallons per minute.[15]

→ **Take shorter, cooler showers**: Take a cue from French and Italian women, with their gorgeously glowy skin, and take shorter (limited to ten minutes), cooler showers. Less time means less water, and less heat means less energy.

→ **Take fewer baths:** This one kind of breaks my heart because I come from a long line of women who read and get drunk in the tub, but it helps to think of soaks as an occasional treat because they use anywhere from twenty-five to fifty gallons, depending on your tub's capacity, while a ten-minute shower with a low-flow showerhead uses only twenty-five gallons.[16]

→ **Install low-flow faucet aerators:** Conventional faucets can use up to three gallons per minute. Low-flow aerators can cut that output by half.[17]

→ **Tackle your toilet:** Flushing a toilet is one of the biggest water hogs in your house, but, ya know, it's gotta happen if you're going to have friends. The average person flushes a toilet five times a day (or fifteen, if you're me), and every flush uses five to seven gallons of precious water.

  • If you own your place, consider a low-flow toilet, which uses 68 percent less water.
  • Only flush the three P's—poo, pee, and (toilet) paper. Avoid tossing tissues, so-called flushable wipes, tampons, nail trimmings, hair, paper towels, condoms, cigarette butts, dental floss, cotton swabs, or whatever else you're trying to shove down the toilet. Not only do these items require a wasteful flush, but they also royally fuck up septic systems and create scary fatbergs that assail sewer systems.[18]

→ **Turn it off:** When you're brushing your teeth, washing dishes, having a dance break, whatever—if you're not actively rinsing off or filling up, turn the tap off. Remember: faucets can flow at three gallons a minute.

→ **Turn it down:** The likelihood of you taking a 140°F shower and enjoying it? Slim-to-none. Most folks have their water heater turned up way too high, so lower it to 120°F, and save some cash (and your skin). If you have an electric water heater, you can also put it on a timer, which can reduce standby energy loss. Fridges and freezers can also benefit from recalibrated temperatures, especially in winter.[19]

→ **Maintain your water heater**: Your water heater is one of the biggest energy users in your home (2,400 kWh annually for a two-person household). Keep it running smoothly with annual draining, and if your water heater is over seven years old, consider swaddling it in an insulation blanket like a giant baby, which can save roughly a thousand pounds of carbon dioxide a year and only costs about $20 to $30 at your hardware store (just make sure the kit is compatible with your water heater).[20]

→ **Hand wash**: Clean delicates and smaller loads of laundry by hand whenever possible.

→ **Full load**: If you must use your dishwashers and washing machines, do so only for full loads. Although I'm sure they're precious to you, your eight white socks or two dinner plates do not merit a full wash cycle of their own.

→ **Collect rainwater**: Sure, this sounds like something fairies would do, but a simple bucket is all you need to catch rainwater to irrigate outdoor plants. Just keep it covered when not collecting to avoid creating a mosquito's dream world.

→ **Regulate that irrigate**: Every year Americans waste close to 18 billion gallons of water (enough to fill the Great Salk Lake twice) on outdoor irrigation. Time-controlled sprinklers may seem like a solid idea but often use 50 percent more water than using a good ol' hose with your good ol' hands. Opt for hand-watering options like hoses and watering cans. Yes, they're old school, but your neighbors will curse you less when they don't have to dodge an errant automatic sprinkler stream on their way to work.[21]

→ **Use undrunk water**: Didn't finish your bedside glass of H_2O? Put it to good use by using it to water your plants.

Heating and Cooling

Most of our residential energy consumption happens when we climate control our spaces—to the tune of 18 percent for cooling and 7 percent for heating.[22] This can vary depending upon your local climate, but taking precautions to ensure your home is well sealed and energy efficient is a great way to save money and prevent resources from literally wafting away. And if you want to turn on Sean Paul's "Temperature" while you read this, here's me giving you an approving, knowing nod that says, "DO IT."

→ **Seal the cracks**: Drafts are a killer when you're trying to climate control your space. Create what experts call a thermal envelope by targeting and sealing drafty culprits:
  - Invest in quality, eco-friendly insulation.
  - Caulk around windows and doors.
  - Install gaskets behind outlets and switches.
  - Make or buy draft dodgers to block drafts typically found under external and internal doors and windows.
  - If you own a home with an attic, insulate the fuck out of it, even if you live in a warmer climate. In the summer, for instance, an attic can get to 150°F, which makes its way down to bake the rest of your space.[23]

→ **Consider windows**: If you own and are in the market for replacements, consider double-glazed windows (which have a pocket of air between the panes that cushions temperatures inside and outside) or options with a low solar heat gain coefficient (SHGC). If you aren't replacing anytime soon, look into low-e coatings and glazes, which are microscopically thin (like, thinner than human hair) and minimize the amount of ultraviolet and infrared light that can pass through glass without compromising visible light.

→ **Block it out**: Curtains and blinds diffuse light in warmer months, keep drafts at bay in cooler seasons, and are a total game killer for Peeping Toms.

→ **Circulate**: Ceiling fans don't cool temps but rather move whatever temperature more seamlessly around your space. Just be sure to turn them off when not in use.

→ **Install a whole-house fan**: These bad boys use up to 90 percent less energy than air conditioners and draw fresh, cool air into the house at night, exhausting hot air through vents.[24]

→ **Passive cooling**: Investigate passive cooling systems like earth tubes, solar chimneys, and reflective roofs. They sound cool because, well, they are and they do.

→ **Solar heating**: While residential solar options can be pricey, if you've got the coin, solar heating systems are excellent for longitudinal cost and energy savings.

→ **Install a smart thermostat**: If you have a central climate system in your home, swap your manual thermostat out in favor of one with smart, programmable options that allow you to limit consumption, often from afar via Wi-Fi, for only when you're at home or you need it. You'll be one step closer to being like my father, Bob, who shows every visitor how he can control his entire house from his iPad.

→ **Air it out**: Whenever possible (temperature and safety of your neighborhood permitting, of course), turn off the appliances, throw open the windows, and let Mother Nature ventilate your home.

→ **Filter**: Replace central system filters monthly, and clean or swap window unit filters every sixty days. Or consider reusable filters. Although more expensive, they recoup their cost in a few years and won't end up in a landfill like traditional air filters that, alas, cannot be recycled.

→ **Kill the lights**: If you've ever tried to change a lit incandescent bulb, you know those suckers get hot as fuck, which can counteract home-cooling efforts. Moreover, keeping any lights blazing in your home when you don't really need them adds peripheral warmth that forces cooling systems to work harder.

→ **Get a better unit**: In a perfect world we'd all cool down via hand fans and mojitos. Alas, a boost from a window unit is sometimes a necessity. If you're in the market, consider secondhand refurbished and/or Energy Star–rated varieties that have eco-modes (that stop whenever desired temperature has been achieved). Only buy the size and BTUs (British thermal units, the per-hour measure of thermal energy) you need, and seal any gaps or cracks around the unit that can let cool air escape.

→ **Go raw**: In warmer months give your stove the night off and your AC a fighting chance by making some no-cook meals (like my Walnut Chorizo Tostadas on page 148—just skip heating up the tortillas).

→ **Bundle up and strip down**: Relying on your climate control to do all the heavy lifting is wasteful as all get-out. If your house is chilly, pop on a cardigan and some slippers. If it's hot in there, well, do as Nelly says, and take off all your clothes.

Plants

You know that new adage about how you shouldn't make out with someone who doesn't own books? No? Just me? Okay, well, the same philosophy applies to a home that doesn't have plants. Not that you'd make out with a home anyway, but . . . okay, starting over. It makes sense that in order to be more thoughtful about the environment, you welcome nature into and around your home. Plants are an economical way to decorate and beautify, clear the air, provide inspiration (and sometimes food), and even save you money on your energy bills, so consider adding real, live (not the plastic crap) plants to every dang room in your house. Following a study into the effects of indoor plants on air pollution, NASA recommends one potted plant per one hundred square feet of space for optimal air clearing. So, go to town, and if someone calls you a "crazy plant person," take that shit as a compliment.[25]

> *Houseplants, a haiku:*
> *O, lil' potted plant,*
> *how you literally breathe*
> *life into my home.*

That's poetry, guys. It's also the truth. Many of us spend 80 to 90 percent of our day indoors, and crummy air quality can lead to a host of health issues (think asthma, heart disease, even cancer).[26] The right florae not only replace CO_2 with life-supporting oxygen but can also dramatically reduce toxins commonly found in new construction buildings and deposited by aerosols and cleaners, such as benzene, formaldehyde, ammonia, xylene, toluene, and trichloroethylene. But how? Easy: science. You see, the biological interaction between plant roots and soil compounds creates micro-organisms that can eat the dangerous air pollutants commonly found indoors. And the appetites of these organisms actually increase relative to the concentration of harmful chemicals in your home's air. That's right—the more crap that's floating in your air, the hungrier they get. Thanks, guys![27]

To get ya started, here's a list of NASA-recommended plants. Bring it to your local nursery or farmers' market, or search Craigslist for rehoming listings and stock up on the good greens:

1. Peace lily
2. Florist's chrysanthemum
3. English ivy
4. Variegated snake plant (I have one of these and it's immortal, even when I accidentally water it with coffee)
5. Re-edged dracaena
6. Cornstalk dracaena
7. Broadleaf lady palm
8. Flamingo lily
9. Devil's ivy
10. Lilyturf

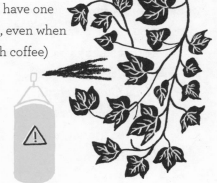

A little note of caution if you have critters: before you bring a plant into your home, make sure they're safe for pets. Some plants, although highly Instagrammable, can be toxic to dogs and cats.

Moreover, I'm not a horticulturalist, and sometimes I have difficulty keeping succulents (billed as "impossible to kill") alive, so I won't be giving you gardening advice. I am, however, going to remind you that growing your own herbs and vegetables (and fruits, where climate and space permit) is rad for soil, your health, your wallet, and your taste buds (four words: fresh basil in winter).

BANG FOR YOUR BARK

According to the USDA Forest Service, strategically planting trees and larger shrubs around your home's exterior can cut air-conditioning needs by 30 percent and heating costs by 20 to 50 percent. The US Department of Energy estimates that just three properly placed trees could save the average household $100 to $250 in energy costs every year.[ix] But what is proper placement?

* Plant deciduous trees (which lose their leaves in winter) on the west side of your home to provide shade in the summer and warming daylight in the winter as they shed their leaves.

* Situate evergreens (which keep their leaves year-round) on the north side of your home to block icy winds, thereby reducing heating needs.

Moreover, trees add tangible value to your home. Homes with mature trees sell for more money ($8,870 more, according to one analysis) and spend less time on the market.[x]

MINIMALISM:
PARE DOWN TO LIVE IT UP

Have you ever been in a home staged for sale? You know what's not in those homes? A whole lotta crap. Realtors go into your space, and before you know it, all the souvenir cups, family caricatures drawn by boardwalk artists, and Mardi Gras beads you so proudly displayed are gone. You see, it's not just because that shit isn't very aesthetically pleasing; it's also because science has proven that less clutter means more serenity. Remember when I mentioned that the average American household contains three hundred thousand–plus items?[28] Experts estimate that Americans waste fifty-five minutes a day just looking for things—that's three thousand hours a year![29] Moreover, all that stuff requires cleaning, a task on which each of us already spends thirty precious days each year.[30] Paring down to only what you use saves time and sanity. And minimalism is a common call to action in this book because the less stuff you have and need, the less strain you put on environmental resources.

Ask yourself six key questions to pare your home down to only the items that bring you peace, productivity, and pleasure:

1. *How often do I use this?* If it's every day or a few times a month, keep it. If you haven't and likely won't use it for six months to a year, donate it.
2. *Do I keep it out of guilt or obligation?* Oh, I know this tale all too well. That unsightly wedding favor (I see you, giant beer stein puff-painted with #JenGetsHarry-ed!) or creepy tribal doll that Aunt Joan brought back for you from Easter Island (that you swear stares at you sometimes) isn't doing you any favors. In fact, they're low-key stressing you the

fuck out. If it's not functional, you don't like it, and you're keeping it out of obligation, determine how important the sentiment is, and either move it into a small mementos box (that you'll put in a storage closet) or donate it. One man's football-shaped phone is another man's treasure, as they say.

3. *Is it important for my job or existence?* Routers can be fugly as hell, but they're kind of essential for staying connected. If something's vital for the work you do or the way you live, keep it.

4. *Does it inspire me?* Not every item in your home needs to have an applied function. Sometimes things are decorative

STORAGE AND CLOWNS

Being the scaredy-cat I am, I've always felt that a jam-packed closet or basement is a more attractive space for a paranormal clown to hide out and eventually haunt my dreams. So if I can't see everything—and I mean EVERYTHING—in those spaces, I know it's time for a cull. As you minimize your home, consider storage spaces as areas to pare down rather than catch-alls for items you cannot muster the urge to purge. Moreover, unless you're stockpiling business inventory or body parts because you're a sociopath, it's pretty unlikely that you actually need storage outside of your home.

Stats show that Americans who rent off-site storage have plenty of other space to utilize if only they got off their duffs and cleared it: 65 percent have a garage, 47 percent have an attic, and 33 percent have a basement. Moreover, self-storage is booming due to our obsession with stuff. There are fifty-three thousand self-storage facilities in America—that's more than all of the Starbucks and McDonald's combined. Research also supports that stored items are often forgotten, and some financial professionals call storage rental a "passive money suck" that can cost $5,000 in just a few years. If you find yourself contemplating enough clutter to merit a rental storage unit, ask yourself if you really need that shit in the first place.[xi]

and provide inspiration, evoke feelings, or just warm your heart. For those things, go with your gut. Marie Kondo touts this method in her uber-popular book, *The Life-Changing Magic of Tidying Up*, urging you to only keep items that "spark joy." It's a great compass for deciding if something stays or goes.[31]

5. ***Do I have duplicates?*** If you've got seven copies of the same beloved book, four different colanders, or three of the same lamp (but you only use two), keep one or two you actually love and use, and donate or sell the rest.

6. ***Do I need to keep it for legal or liability reasons?*** I don't want to make you a paranoid hoarder, but sometimes you need to keep things for no other reason than to protect yourself. Parts of your rental that have fallen apart that you'll need to return when you move out, legal documents, receipts for reimbursements or big-ticket items, personal identification docs, some memorabilia or keepsakes (which will protect you from epic guilt trips). Determine what those are, and set aside a small folder or box for them.

MOVING ON UP

It's a truth almost universally recognized that moving sucks. It especially stinks for the friends you've tapped twelve times to hulk your armoire down three flights of stairs in exchange for a six-pack and salty pizza. Luckily, now that you give a shit, when you do move you'll hopefully have way less stuff to haul. Moreover, moving doesn't require a million oft-discarded boxes and packing tape. Many areas boast rentable reusable box services that, for a nominal fee, will deliver sturdy, roomy tubs with lids to your home, where you can fill 'em up and, once you're moved to your next location, they'll retrieve the empties. The feeling of not having to loiter in the grocery store parking lot looking for boxes? Priceless.

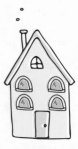

OUTFITTING YOUR ECO-HOME: ROOM BY ROOM

Now that you've established a bomb-ass in-home waste-reduction system, embraced energy-efficient practices, and purged unwanted clutter, it's time to go room by room, MTV *Cribs* style. Mind you, this isn't an exhaustive listing of every room in every house (if you have an in-home bowling alley or movie theater, for example, I don't have sections for those, but please invite me over) or a prescription for exactly and only what you can or should have to be eco-friendly. It's up to you to take this guidance and apply it as you see fit to your own household.

Entryway

The entryway to your home—be it a sprawling foyer or a humble ledge by the door—should be a welcoming space that also helps you keep your shit together so you're not that person who's constantly locked out of her house, eye makeup running here and there, with no wallet, and a half-eaten granola bar in her pocket (nods head). "But Ashlee, how is this eco-friendly?" Well, for one, entryways are often the intersection of the essentials we need to be productive human beings (keys, wallet, phone) and pesky clutter (piled-up mail and shoes) that, when left unmanaged, can make your day hella stressful. And because minimalism is an underlying ethos that helps us embrace more sustainable habits, it makes sense that we're starting literally at the beginning: your front door.

MAIL CULL

Love letters, cards from your grandma, unexpected checks—some snail mail is just freaking awesome. Unwelcomed paper clutter in the form of the one hundred billion pieces of junk mail distributed annually in the United States, however, is not.[32] Here's the skinny: the average American receives about forty-one pounds of junk mail per year (for an annual total of five million TONS), 44 percent of which goes straight to the landfill.[33] Junk mail not only contributes to deforestation but also annoyingly makes you more susceptible to buying shit you don't need. Marketers operate on the principle that it takes seven impressions before you'll buy their product or service, so their paper-based pursuit is relentless.[34]

Here are some simple steps that make the landfill pariah of unsolicited mail easily avoidable:[35]

→ **Go paperless**: This may sound like a giant duh, but take a few minutes to ensure any accounts that have attendant statements (bank, credit card, loans, mortgage—you get the idea) are set to paperless billing whenever possible. You'd think this would be the default in our modern world, but many companies still require an explicit opt-in for paperless billing and communique.

→ **Get on the list**: Curb unsolicited mail by getting on "do not mail" lists. There are many sites that will help you cut through the noise, but you will likely need to visit or contact a few to cover your bases:
  • CatalogChoice.org: Search for individual companies and

organizations and access opt-out instructions.

- OptOutPrescreen.com: Reduce credit card offers.
- DMACHOICE.org: Opt out of catalogs, magazines, credit offers, and any other "offers," even from companies with which you've never done business.
- InfoCision: This is a telemarketing company that manages marketing lists for clients. Call or email to request removal. Bonus: fewer telemarketer calls interrupting your binge watching.
- YellowPagesOptOut: Decline phone book delivery. Remember those?

→ **Simplify subscriptions**: Listen, I write for, read, and love me some print magazines and newspapers. That said, most of us don't need or have the bandwidth to skim fifteen new periodicals coming our way each month. I personally went down to two subscriptions, and when I'm done enjoying them, I share with friends, leave at the gym for others to peruse, and even donate to after-school programs and homeless shelters so they never hit the recycle bin without some solid reuse.

→ **Give strategically**: Philanthropy is truly a cornerstone of a life well lived. That said, many charities sell smaller donors' contact info to other orgs because little donations, while great, don't help them recoup their costs. Charity Navigator recommends making larger gifts to fewer organizations rather than smaller gifts to many. This maximizes your contribution and lands your name on fewer lists.[36]

→ **Guard your info**: The less your personal info is out there, the less it can be exploited. Whenever possible, remove your mailing address from checks, email signatures, social media accounts (really, guys, have Lifetime movies taught you nothing?), petitions, and other unnecessary places.

These steps should dramatically reduce the amount of unwanted mail you receive, but be patient. Mailings are usually prepared in advance, so it can take three to six months to see serious results. For the junk that still creeps in, consider reusing the envelopes as scrap paper for notes and recycling appropriately when you've exhausted other conceivable uses.

HELP THY NEIGHBOR

Pay it forward and help an elderly, non-tech savvy relative or neighbor get off junk mail lists. Why? Seniors are disproportionately bombarded with junk mail, receiving an average twenty-five pieces a week to a younger person's fifteen. Moreover, 40 percent of elderly persons have been victimized by fraud, and an influx of junk mail received is a good indication that scammers also have access to their information. A few minutes of your time will help alleviate their stress, and you'll probably get to hear incredible stories and eat some butterscotch candies because older people totally rule.[xii]

Living Room

Perhaps the most catch-all room of any home, the living room serves many masters. Instead of boring you with an overly prescriptive list of what you should and shouldn't have in this room (that's really up to you and how your family lives), I'm instead going to show you how to appoint it and the rest of your home like a goddamn green-leaning boss.

THINK SECONDHAND FIRST

In 2009 the EPA noted that furniture accounted for 9.8 million tons (4.1 percent) of all American household waste. Furniture is also the number-one least-recycled item in a home for a variety of reasons ranging from simply not knowing what the hell to do with something to dumpers being really fucking lazy. Furniture's also expensive. In 2015 Americans were estimated to have spent $121.7 billion on new furnishings, the production of which guzzles tremendous resources and creates serious emissions.[37]

I evangelize about the benefits of buying secondhand like a sweaty preacher on a balmy Sunday morning. For one, resale is the very embodiment of the sustainable principles of reducing, reusing, and recycling. Moreover, while secondhand stuff wrongly gets a bad rap as being in disrepair, dated, or contaminated, the truth is that resale items can be sturdier, range from timeless to trendy, and are easily restored to their original glory with a little clever elbow grease or a quick repair. You see, we're so often told that if we are seeking better quality, we require something brand new. But that's just a marketing ploy. Up until the 1930s, items were built to last nearly a lifetime. However, the post-Depression American desire for job security and a near-obsessive belief that prosperity was best communicated through new things created a manufacturing approach that experts call "planned obsolescence," or the making of things with an intentional artificially limited use life. If you're thinking this is a dirty trick, it is. Kind of. The origins of which were decently well intentioned—make shoddier items so consumers need to buy more, thus creating jobs and reducing rampant Depression-era unemployment. However, today manufacturers make it nearly impossible to avoid this "contrived durability" by phasing out repair options (when was the last time you saw a brick-and-mortar television repair shop?) while simultaneously creating faultier products. We're left with little choice but to buy a new one because you can only go so long without a working fridge. The point here is that built-in obsolescence, buttressed by the rise of "fast" manufacturing, shatters the commonly held belief that newer is better.[38]

Moreover, used doesn't always mean used within an inch of its life. I've scored barely touched, pristine-condition, discontinued (and, thus, in high demand) designer furnishings and duds for a fraction of the retail price. All because I was willing to wait a minute and do a little hunting. So whether you're outfitting your home with furniture and décor, buying a set of wheels, or revamping your wardrobe, think secondhand first. I've gotten to the point where I love the patience, pursuit, and interesting secondhand-item histories so much that buying new has almost entirely lost its luster.

SECONDHAND SCORES

The options for resale furnishings and goods are endless and ever changing, but here are some of my favorites:

✳ *Craigslist:* Simply the best option if you're searching for something specific or discontinued (hi, West Elm Midcentury Marble Coffee Table) and don't want to travel all over creation to get it. Hot tip: always scour the "free" section before hitting the pay-for-play listings.

✳ *Freecycle:* A solid option for the less choosy, more penny-pinching among us.

✳ *Local brick-and-mortar resale/charity shops:* Fuck yes to these places. I sashay in and feel like Holly Golightly at Tiffany's. Selections change often, prices are usually more reasonable than vintage stores, and many purchases benefit charity. So ask around, check out reviews, and live that resale truth.

✳ *The curb:* Or the alleys/curbs of way more affluent areas. It's baffling, but even the wealthiest among us are not too high-falootin' to put their cast-offs on the street. And bless 'em for that, because that's how I got my first DVD player. Rescuing furniture from the curb is one of my favorite activities and that makes me a cheap date. Hot tip: check the "free" section of Craigslist in your area because people often list when and where they're going to abandon total treasures (called "curb alerts").

WHEN YOU'VE GOTTA BUY NEW

Sometimes our needs are so immediate or specific that we must resort to buying new. And when that happens, instead of flogging yourself, stay attentive to the following to ensure your money is supporting an ethical, sustainable product that will withstand the test of time (and your toddler's tantrums).

→ **Do your homework**: Before you shop, check out the Sustainable Furnishings Council's directory of member companies committed to greener products and manufacturing practices.

→ **Opt for multifunction**: A towering computer desk serves one purpose, while a solid wood table can grow with your needs from computer desk to dining space to workbench. A streamlined dresser, for instance, can morph easily into an entertainment center, clothing storage, and a baby changing table with a few small tweaks. The more functions a piece can serve, the better the likelihood that it'll grow with you.

→ **Opt for natural, sustainable materials**: Responsibly harvested wood (like fast-growing bamboo), metal, glass, organic cotton and linen upholstery, recycled plastic, and reclaimed materials, when paired with sound construction, all mean that your new furniture will reach heirloom-quality status even after decades of use.

→ **Buy untreated or unfinished**: Avoid toxic off-gassing by purchasing furniture that has been naturally treated or left untreated.

→ **Look at longevity**: The most eco-friendly items are those that don't end up in a landfill, so whenever possible, repair, repurpose, and purchase with durability in mind. Look for lifetime guarantees, repair options, and warranties, which are good signs a company is committed to making your relationship with that chair or desk last forever.

→ **Demand transparency**: Many symbols and certifications exist that show a company gives a shit about workers and the environment. Here are a few to keep in mind:

- Forest Stewardship Council (FSC) Chain of Custody: Certifies and monitors sustainable wood harvesting.
- Greenguard: Minimizes toxic materials in furnishings. And if you think this sounds crunchy, design trailblazers like Herman Miller and Knoll make this cert a priority in many of their offerings.
- Business and Institutional Furniture Manufacturers Association (BIFMA) Certifications: Third parties ensure manufacturing processes positively impact the environment and human health.
- Green Seal Certified: Involves thirty-three sustainability standards that cover over four hundred different kinds of products.
- Global Organic Textile/Latex Standards (GOTS and GOLS, respectively): The gold standards for soft materials, which certify that at least 95 percent of an item is made of certified organic materials and that certain chemistries are prohibited entirely (even for that other 5 percent), including polyurethane foam and fire retardants. Moreover, businesses must adhere to environmentally friendly practices, including shipping, waste disposal, and printing.

→ **Support small and local**: Wherever you live, I'd bet that there are local craftspeople who make baller-looking, durable furnishings. Explore those options to cut down on shipping emissions and support your neighborhood artisan.

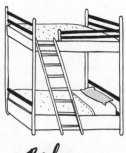

Bedrooms

Cue the slow jams, everyone, because we're talking about the sexiest room in the house. That's right, it's the (bow chicka wow wow) bedroom. As with all the areas in your home, let's think about the purpose, shall we? In no particular order, bedrooms are for: sleeping, devouring a good book, spooning your pets against their will, convalescing when you're sick, and hanky-pankying till the break of dawn. With those activities in mind, a bedroom really doesn't require much equipment (looking at you, flat-screen TV), and that's good because it's supposed to be a restful space, and more stuff = less zen.

OUTFITTING YOUR BEDROOM

Although a bed is a pretty essential element for a bedroom, how you frame that bed is up to you. The hardcore collegiate among us have been known to rock a mattress on the floor, while others have a four-poster California king with two box springs. There's a happy medium somewhere in there, and that's kind of up to you, but here are some tips for furnishing your bedroom for restful elegance without a lot of fuss:

→ **Keep it simple**: A room where you're mostly passed out doesn't need a lot of furniture. A bed frame, side table, light source, and dresser are all you really need. Any extra items just require more clutter, cleaning, and money.

→ **Skip the box spring**: Nothing strikes fear in the hearts of friends asked to help you move like a box spring and a fourth-floor walk-up. They're difficult to maneuver, even harder to dispose of, and aren't even really necessary. Opt for a bed frame like a platform bed that doesn't require a box spring.

→ **Buy secondhand**: Even if you're squeamish about getting softer surfaces resale, bed frames, night tables, lamps, and other solid furnishings are cheaper and more sustainable when they're secondhand. Refer back to the Secondhand Stores sidebar on page 60 for more guidance.

→ **Use curtains**: Window shades and curtains effectively block sleep-disrupting light while also offering eco-friendly climate control (and privacy for your gettin' down).

→ **No TV**: I'm going to seem very uptight for suggesting this, but Americans already watch about thirty-five-plus hours of television per week. Why would you want to sacrifice reparative, restful sleep time for an energy-guzzling device that allows advertisers and disturbing images to invade your dreams? Need more convincing? According to one study, couples who had a TV in the bedroom apparently had sex half as often as those who didn't. You hear that? That's the sound of every man in America throwing his television out the window.[39]

SLEEP ON IT

In addition to spending 90 percent of our time indoors, we spend 25 percent of our lives catching ZZZs. So it makes sense that we'd want to ensure that our bed, the place where we're facedown roughly fifty-six hours each week, is cozy, safe, and as sustainable as possible.[40]

Mattresses

The average mattress can contain a toxic cocktail of petrochemicals, known carcinogens, and flame-retardants that can cause health issues and are never able to be safely assimilated back into the environment.

Moreover, even if you sleep on your mattress solo, you're never really alone. WUT? Yeah, your mattress, which houses your shed skin flakes, sweat, and oil over time, is a fave hangout for hundreds of eight-legged darlings known as dust mites. This isn't abnormal (we all shed skin, and that's a mite's fave meal), unique to traditional mattresses (eco-beds get dust mites too), or dangerous (they can cause allergies for some but aren't going to harm you), but after ten years those suckers can really add up, signaling that it might be

NOTHING REALLY MATTRESS

Mattresses are some of the most difficult items to off-load. Not a weekend goes by that I don't see those saggy, suspiciously stained bastards out on the curb. So be extra thoughtful about (1) whether you need a new one and (2) the next one you buy. Moreover, you can easily extend the life of your existing mattress with a few easy fixes:

✳ *Vacuum and flip it regularly to keep dust mites to a minimum and prevent one-sided wear.*

✳ *Invest in a low-toxicity cover to prevent your cooties from seeping into the mattress.*

✳ *Shore up a sagging foundation with a reclaimed wood board.*

✳ *Add an eco-friendly topper if you need extra squishiness in your slumber.*

And if you must bid your bed adieu, give it a proper sendoff and avoid the alley. Many charities and folks on Craigslist and Freecycle will gladly take it, and responsible mattress recycling services are available for a small fee.

the time to invest in a new, eco-friendly version. And while you're at it, consider your pillows as well, as they can fall prey to the same buggy fate.[41]

Luckily, the eco-mattress and pillow game is booming and brimming with options. Keep an eye out for materials like 100 percent natural latex (which is safer than latex blends, which often contain petroleum-based polyurethane) and organic and pesticide-free cotton, which can be gentler on the environment and safer for your health. Because few of us are textile experts, it's important to keep your eyes peeled for some heavy-hitter certifications so you can feel more confident that what you're buying is devoid of toxic garbage and is truly sustainably produced:

→ **GOTS and GOLS,** as covered on page 62.

→ **Oeko-Tex Standard 100**: Sets limits for volatile organic compounds (VOC) emissions, such as formaldehyde, and prohibits the use of dangerous flame retardants and dyes.

→ **Oeko-Tex Standard 1000**: Mandates that companies meet strict specifications regarding wastewater treatment and waste air emissions; use eco-friendly technologies, energy, and materials; demonstrate workplace hygiene and safety; and comply with prohibitions on child and forced labor, livable wages, and regulated work hours.

→ **USDA Certified Biobased**: Certifies that a product or package contains a verified amount of renewable biological ingredients.

→ **Formaldehyde Free UL**: Through audits and sample testing, validates that a product does not contain formaldehyde or precursors.

→ **OCS100 Organic Content Standard**: Ensures proper tracking of organic material from its source to the finished product.

→ **Forest Stewardship Council® (FSC)/Rainforest Alliance Chain of Custody**: Ensures that natural latex meets rigorous environmental, social, and economic criteria designed to protect lands, ecosystems, and workers.

→ **Made Safe**: Certifies that a product has been made with ingredients not known or suspected to cause human health harm.[42]

DOWN WITH DOWN

I'm an ethical vegan, so I don't wear or use animal products on principle. I'm also constantly chilly and live in a turn-of-the-century apartment in Chicago. Although down and wool are natural materials popularly used in cold-weather clothes and bedding, the methods by which they are harvested cause serious suffering for innocent animals. Contrary to what we're led to believe, sheep shearing and feather plucking aren't gentle processes. They're traumatic, causing pain and sometimes death, and even if the animals survive one or repeated harvests, they're slaughtered once their wool- and feather-bearing prime has passed. Thankfully, innovative sustainable materials exist that are durable, warm as heck, and spare our fine fleecy and feathered friends from unnecessary harm. Look for widely available down alternatives, cotton flannel, polyester fleece, wool-like felt made from recycled materials, and even upcycled options when selecting toasty textiles. And if you must buy down or wool, consider doing so secondhand.[xiii]

Linens

Some of the same standards apply to bedding, but you needn't run out and buy all new sheets to give a shit. Assess what you have, and if you need to bring some additions into the mix, consider the following options:

→ Bed linens made from natural, breathable materials like organic cotton, bamboo, hemp, wood pulp (also called Lyocell, Tencel, and Legna), and, my personal favorite, linen (which is sustainable as hell, lasts for years, and prevents night sweats while still keeping you cozy all year round).

→ Consider secondhand blankets and afghans, which are often restored to their grandma-cozy glory with a hearty hot-water wash.

→ Keep things simple by only having two sets of sheets per bed, following the one-in-use, one-in-storage philosophy.

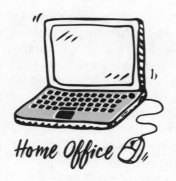

Home Office

I have a confession to make: one of my favorite stress relievers back in the day was to go to a posh stationery store and drop major Benjamins on greeting cards, cool gel pens, glittery notebooks, and other stuff I didn't really need. Like most people, I get that "I'm starting fresh!" rush when I have new supplies. But we don't need all that stuff. I'm not saying you can't have a funky notebook or favorite pen, but if you're a Post-it addict or someone who prints and chucks documents constantly, let's explore some habits that better align with the Give a Shit lifestyle.

As with any room in your house, the place where you cook up hot, multimillion-dollar ideas (or just pulse a stress squeezer as you rewrite a sternly worded email to your lazy coworker for the fiftieth time) should be clutter-free. Why? Blank space just begs to be filled with brilliant ideas. Now, I recognize that not everyone works this way, but even the biggest pack rat can benefit from the occasional office clear-out. And these principles can be applied to any work location, not just the home-based variety:

→ **Go digital**: Embrace apps that digitize receipts and invoices (Receiptmate) and business cards (Haystack), organize notes (Evernote), create legally binding signatures sans printing (HelloSign, DocuSign), sync calendars and to-do lists (WunderList), collaborate on documents (Google Docs), and do basically anything else you'd normally do with or on paper.

→ **Regulate papers**: Refuse receipts or, if you must have them (for higher-ticket items you may return), opt for electronic. You see, most receipts are made from thermal paper, which, when entering the recycling system, contaminates it with BPA. So refuse them if at all possible. Manuals and warranties for larger, more expensive items can usually be accessed online, so you don't need to keep the gigantic paper versions around.

→ **Supply sustainably**: Refillable pens, low-waste writing tools like chalk, dry erase boards, and colored pencils (which handily replace highlighters), recycled and compostable paper, and

PEN FOR YOUR THOUGHTS?

According to the EPA, Americans toss 1.6 billion disposable pens each year. If you're into math, that's about two pens every year for each person in the United States (which is weird because when was the last time you actually finished a pen?). Investing in a refillable pen is not only awesome for the environment but also makes you look like a serious businessperson à la a Cary Grant film. Think about it: you'll be low-key saving the planet while also yelling "Where's my special pen?" throughout the office in a cantankerous voice like a cool old police detective everyone fears and respects.[xiv]

paper clips (which serve the same purpose as staples but are reusable) alleviate environmental burden whilst still helping you get the job done.

→ **Share resources**: While back-to-school is practically a national holiday in America, brand-spankin'-new supplies simply aren't necessary for success. Assess what you have at home, and if you need something, ask neighbors if they have extras. Consider holding a resource swap where everyone brings and swaps their extra supply inventory (this works well with intermittent-use items like graphing calculators, 3D printers, and even certain musical instruments), buying secondhand, or checking out from your local library.

→ **Police your printing**: If you must use a printer, consider using both sides of recycled paper, recycled and refillable ink and toner cartridges, using "draft" mode and printing only in black and white to extend cartridge life, and reducing margin settings to use less paper.

→ **Start stripping**: Those eyes in the darkness of your home aren't bats; they're the glowing buttons of something more menacing: energy vampires. Because an estimated 5 to 10 percent of household energy (and 1 percent of carbon dioxide emissions) is wasted through standby consumption, a smart-power strip will shut down power to products with standby modes so you don't have to go around the house unplugging everything like a Luddite.[43]

→ **Skip the screensaver**: No one really gleans inspo from your "hang in there" cat screensaver, so put that shit on energy-saving mode.

→ **Opt for laptops**: If you have a choice, laptops are 80 percent more energy efficient than desktop computers and, depending upon models, can use up to a third less energy.[44]

Bathrooms

Let's think for a minute about the actual purpose of a bathroom. Despite what my candor in this book may lead you to think, I actually do not like talking about human bathroom functions. Like, I hate it. Perhaps it's the one holdout from my pretty genteel southern upbringing, but I'm definitely not the kind of girl whose heart is warmed by fart jokes on a first (or seventeenth) date. That said, as with any room in your home, we gotta get real about the primary purpose. A bathroom is for human elimination (and a decent amount of reading or texting during, let's be honest), getting clean, relaxing soaks, bathing kiddos and/or pets (if you've got 'em), and general grooming routines. Sure, sometimes the bathroom is for in-shower karaoke or steamy lovemaking, but unless you're a breathing reenactment of the movie 9½ *Weeks* (in which case, #jealous), I highly doubt you're going to need a sex bench in your powder room.

At its core a bathroom should be functional and serene so you (and guests) can get in, do your thing with ease, and get out in the world clean and confident. A minimalist bathroom only really needs:

→ Two towels and two washcloths per person (one of each stored while the other is being used; consider cotton, bamboo, hemp, or linen)

→ One washable or reusable (like bamboo) bathmat

→ Two hand/guest towels (one stored while the other is being used)

→ One washable shower curtain liner: these liners can be washed with your regular laundry, which keeps them mold- and stink-free, and are IMHO way less alarming feeling when they graze and cling to your naked body in the shower.

→ One washable shower curtain

→ One squeegee (if you have glass shower doors, as opposed to a curtain)

→ Water-saving showerhead

→ Drain catcher/plug (to catch hair, which you can compost later)

→ One small trash can with lid (more on this later)

BUTTS ABOUT IT

It's a wonder that someone as squeamish as I am about bodily functions is writing about things that clean your bum, but here we are. Easy swaps on the porcelain throne actually make a big difference.

✳ **Swap your roll:** *Opt for recycled toilet paper (no, that doesn't mean it's recycled from used toilet paper, guys) with a compostable core. Most bundles are wrapped in plastic, but certain hotel, industrial supply outlets, and home delivery services sell individual rolls wrapped in paper, which can be composted or recycled and, thus, are more sustainable.*

✳ **Consider a bidet:** *It sounds fancy and high-tech, but bidets have been all the rage in other countries for a long-ass time. They require little water (by eliminating the use of toilet paper, bidets actually use less water), get ya clean as a whistle, cut down on paper waste, and are easy to install, even if you rent. And if you do have a bidet, it's a good idea to have a roll of TP around for guests who get freaked by water spontaneously squirting on their badonkadonk.*

→ One pump bottle or bar of castile soap for hand washing (skip the antibacterial—I elaborate as to why on page 216)

→ Homemade air freshener and/or cute box of matches (skip the synthetic stuff)

→ Two rolls of recycled toilet paper with compostable core (one stored while the other is used)

→ Bidet, if that's your bag

→ Simple hooks for towels and robes

TOWEL TALK

Although I sort of admire the dedication of people who have, like, three hundred pristine white towels in their linen closets, unless you're running a bed and breakfast, you really don't need all that noise in your life. Remember, you're trying to ease the burden not only on the environment but also on yourself. Bath linens require washing, which sucks up energy and time, so assess what your household actually needs. As a general rule of thumb, each member of your home should have two bath towels and two washcloths (or none, if they don't use 'em), meaning that when one is in use the other can be washed or stored. This philosophy also lessens the likelihood that they'll end up on the floor in a damp heap of sadness. If you're currently using a fresh towel after every shower, it's time for an intervention, friend: you're already (hopefully?) clean when you exit the shower or bath, so using the same towel for a few days ain't gonna contaminate you.

Hand towels are pretty essential because, well, you've gotta wash and dry your hands. I recommend having two public-facing (meaning they're decently presentable and don't look like they were used to clean up a murder scene) cloth hand towels, abiding by the same one-in-use, one-in-storage principle. I don't know when people started using fancy paper napkins for hand drying, but cut the shit, guys. I'm pretty sure you're not running a Five-Star resort, and I can't think of anything more wasteful.

We're not looking for perfection here either. If you have a still-very-useful, washable IKEA bathmat (points to self), by golly, keep a good thing going. You don't need to run out and buy a bushel of new things to give a shit.

TOWEL TRANSFORMATION

We all have janky towels that probably shouldn't see the light of day, but boy they've seen some life. The black towel that tells the tale of when you tried to bleach your hair Khaleesi white? The beige hand towel permanently stained an unsettling Pepto Bismol pink from the time you vomited up an entire bottle of Petit Syrah on your floor? It's not the towels' fault, but you're just not about that life anymore. Well, there is a place where janky towels can have their well-deserved happily ever after: the animal shelter! Ya see, with all the spills and thrills adorable adoptable critters get up to, most shelters will gladly take your old towels (and blankets and sheets!). Wash 'em, bring 'em over, and bless up that your trash can be a little kitten's treasure!

(TRASH)CAN YOU NOT?

You'll notice that the bathroom is the only place I suggest you have an actual trash can. This is more for other peeps than for you. I say this because you don't want guests coming over and having a mild panic attack because there's no place for them to dispose of a feminine hygiene product or hypodermic needle (kidding). A small, preferably metal trash can with a lid is discreet enough to not be an eyesore while still hitting the message home that "this ain't no trashy home." I personally do not use liners in my trashcan because it so rarely gets used, and when it does, I simply give it a wash in the sink. But if liners are helpful in your transition to being more low waste, be sure you're using biodegradable versions that are minimally packaged and that you reuse or repurpose them whenever possible.

ONE WORD: FATBERG

If you're eating, stop now. You'll notice that a Give a Shit bathroom does not contain facial tissues, so-called flushable wipes, or paper towels. This is not only because they're wasteful as hell but also because when flushed they amass with other foreign matter to create ginormous congealed lumps of sewer-clogging crazy called fatbergs. Don't believe me? London recently wrangled a 130-ton fatberg that cost $130 million a month to dismantle. So swap wet wipes (which, sure, can be flushed, but so can a child's flip-flop) for recycled toilet paper or a bidet, tissues for cloth handkerchiefs (much more dignified), and paper towels for reusable cloths so you don't assist in the creation of a real-life reenactment of The Blob. For the purists out there: flush only the three P's (I'm too much of a lady to reiterate, but you get the idea).[xv]

Laundry Room

As certain as death and taxes, in every life at least a little laundry must be done. According to our friends at the Bureau of Labor Statistics, Americans spend eight hours a week doing laundry-related activities, with women logging eighteen minutes to men's totally not shocking four minutes a day. Here's what you can do to make doing laundry easier for you and peachier for the planet:[45]

→ **Hand wash**: Contrary to popular belief, your underwear doesn't need a cycle all its own. Whenever possible, wash things by hand.

→ **Chill out**: Did you know that 90 percent of energy used during a conventional wash cycle is expended on heating the water? Unless you just got back from a mud run, a standard load will still get clean as a whistle washed on cold.[46]

→ **Fill it up**: Unless your signature color is crisp white, separating lights and darks into their own loads is a waste of time and energy. This will also make it easier for you to do full loads of laundry and do them less often.

→ **Freeze**: This is going to sound wild, but placing clothes and accessories like jeans, sweaters, pantyhose and tights, and stinky shoes in your freezer (in a paper bag) helps to remove odor-causing bacteria, preserve fabric strength and color-fastness (because you're not washing constantly), and even prevent shedding.

→ **Air dry**: Drying racks and clotheslines are gentler-on-clothes (no shrinkage!) alternatives to running a hot, energy-guzzling dryer.

→ **Dump dryer sheets**: Loaded with often animal-tested toxic chemicals and fragrances, dryer sheets are wasteful and ridic. Plus, they're guaranteed to secretly stow away in your pants only to make an embarrassing appearance on your ass during your work presentation. Dryer balls, like those made from wool or vegan alternatives, naturally remove static from clothes and can be reused for a long-ass time (and if they're natural material, composted thereafter).[47]

→ **Freshen naturally**: Consider homemade air freshener and essential oils (a little tapped into a dryer ball works wonders). Moreover, if you have wooden shelves in your closet or drawers in your dresser, tap a little essential oil (I love cedarwood, lavender, and eucalyptus) right into the wood (being careful not to get the oil on your clothes) to freshen garments.

→ **Choose cleaner cleaners**: Advertisements tell us that we need pretreaters, stain removers, detergents, bleach and oxygenating whitening potions, scent boosters, fabric softeners, dryer sheets, wrinkle reducers, spray starch, and a host of other heavily fragranced and packaged crap to get our clothes clean. Don't buy into the hype. Streamline your routine with the home care recipes in this book, or if DIY's not your bag, opt for minimally packaged (powders and concentrates over liquids), cruelty-free, environmentally friendly, natural options. Peep my favorites at ashleepiper.com/LBB.

→ **Bag it up**: Prevent microplastics from contaminating waterways by washing synthetic items like polyester in specially designed bags that block plastic and foreign matter from weaseling their way into drinking water and rivers.

→ **Wise up on wrinkles**: If you're the type who needs to look pressed on the daily, hanging and smoothing clothes while they're still warm from the dryer minimizes wrinkles without having to fire up the iron. When you need to look crisp as fuck, an energy-efficient iron (skip the starch) or steamer is a great alternative to dry cleaning. Speaking of which . . .

→ **Bye, dry cleaners**: Janice down the street at my local dry cleaner is gonna be pissed when she reads this, but dry cleaning is not only expensive (an average of $500 per year for the average American), but even the "green" ones use toxic, often animal-tested cleaning agents that can pollute waterways.[48] A great way to bypass the dry cleaner is by purchasing items that don't require dry cleaning in the first place. If you do have more delicate items, consider hand washing first.

→ **Opt for energy efficient**: Whether you buy new or refurbished, Energy Star–certified washers and electric dryers are 25 percent and 20 percent more efficient, respectively, than standard models (a certified clothes washer alone can save up to $490 over ten years). You'll also use approximately 45 percent less water. Many electric companies will also offer you a rebate for purchasing energy-efficient models.[49]

Kitchen

You may have heard through the fake-news grapevine that cooking and eating sustainably means that you need to overhaul your kitchen, learn how to sprout things, and become an expert fermenter, whatever that means. Au contraire, mon frère. Although you may want to invest in *some* special items that make you feel like a green queen (or king), you certainly don't have to—and none of these shifts need to be made immediately or expensively (most of the items, especially metal and glass items, can be found second-hand for a song). Above all, a happy kitchen is an easy-to-navigate one, featuring only the items you use frequently, stowed appropriately for that ever-elusive but oh-so-wonderful clear countertop feel. If you don't regularly make waffles, bake bread, or pressure cook, eschew single-purpose counter hogs, and outfit your galley with only the items you absolutely need. Mark Bittman, a food writer

THROW IN THE TOWEL

First, the bad news: paper towels are incredibly wasteful. Not only do they account for an estimated 254 million tons of global trash every year, but they also require significant resources (seventeen trees and twenty thousand gallons of water to produce just one ton). Oh, and although they may seem inexpensive, people who hit their paper towel habit hard end up spending upward of $600 per year. Let that soak in.

The good news? Paper towels are incredibly easy to sustainably swap. Get some absorbent cotton, hemp, or linen cloths (or, if you really give a shit, fashion some by cutting up old tees, button-downs, or sheets), use them as you would paper towels, and wash with your usual laundry. Cheap, cheerful, and tidy, this is one of the simplest shifts you'll ever make. And the eco-payoff is fab: if every US household used just one less seventy-sheet roll of paper towels, we'd save 544,000 trees, forty thousand tons of waste, and $1.4 million in landfill dumping fees.[xvi]

of global renown, says he creates gourmet meals in a microscopic kitchen with a well-edited (read: super-spare) arsenal of kitchen tools. If he can do it, you can too.[50]

MAKE THE KITCH YOUR BITCH

When paring down and reappointing your kitchen, ask yourself these questions:

→ *What meals do I make most frequently?* For instance, I have a smoothie pretty much every morning, so a high-speed blender is a must for me. If your afternoon cup of tea is essential to your well-being, then by George, get a teakettle that brings you joy.

→ *How often do I actually entertain?* Dinner parties are awesome, but unless you're hosting them every month, you probably don't need twenty place settings, crystal goblets, and a bazillion serving vessels. These items can easily be picked up secondhand or borrowed from a neighbor when the urge to Ina Garten strikes.

→ *What's the lowest-waste version I'm willing to try for this?* I mentioned earlier how I'm a coffee addict. I, like 27 percent of Americans, also used to have one of those K-cup coffee machines that produce ten times the solid waste than a standard drip brewer, most of which isn't recyclable. Caffeine at the touch of a button was fun, but I found that switching to a no-waste French press (no filters and I simply compost the grounds when I'm done) required little extra effort and produced the same tasty slurp while also significantly cutting down on waste, cost, and hassle (I never have to run out for pods or filters). Review your culinary rituals to determine low-sacrifice ways to make them simpler and more sustainable.[51]

→ *How many do I actually need?* Unless you're running a catering business, you probably don't need fourteen cake stands. Same goes for saucepans, colanders, and anything else in your kitchen (and life).

→ *Do current items have other uses?* What did chefs do before the garlic press, spiralizer, and citrus zester, guys? Easy. They made do with other items that worked pretty darn well. A quality set of kitchen knives can replace graters, zesters, presses, and a host of other niche accoutrements. A metal colander, for instance, can strain pasta and broths, sift flours, wash farmers' market finds, and mash potatoes. Get creative!

→ *Is it timeless?* Have you ever been out to eat? Yeah, me too. It's a fun time. You know what pretty much every dining establishment, whether fancy or casual, has in common? A simple set of white plates. Now, I'm not saying you can only have plain stuff, but I encourage you to consider the longevity of the items you bring into your abode.

→ *Will it last?* The materials and craftsmanship of our home's most-used implements can significantly increase their life-span, thereby saving us money and time. Natural materials and solid construction usually mean longer use. Consider a cast-iron skillet versus a more cheaply made Teflon-type version. Sure, the latter is lighter and costs less upfront, but with a little maintenance, the cast-iron will outlive you. And as with any new purchases, opt for lifetime warranties and repair options. Cutco Knives, Pampered Chef cookware, and certain Le Creuset products boast lifetime guarantees, which will keep you cookin' through the decades.

If you're the type who needs a checklist to jump-start your journey, you're in luck, because I just so happen to have one (removes wad of paper from bra). I recommend the following essentials when folks are looking to cut down on kitchen clutter and still eat amazing food, but every household's culinary and dining needs are different, so you do you. One person's panini press is another person's eyesore.

NOT GROSS. PROMISE.

I get the natural nervousness that may arise when considering secondhand kitchen swag. It feels a little like you're getting regurgitated food, but I can assure you that's not the case. My primary consideration for buying secondhand is how clean I can get something. I generally advise against buying plastic (because, well, plastic) and wooden cooking items secondhand because they often hold bacteria and are difficult to sterilize. The exception here for me is an amazing wooden potato bowl from the late 1800s that I inherited and now use to handsomely present fruit. Metal and glass items, however, are easy to find secondhand and can be restored to their original glory with a little elbow grease. Besides, it's kind of cool to think that a good cleaning is often the only thing standing between you and a soup pot that has some dope stories to tell.

Cooking

- Wood (like bamboo) or metal cooking utensils
- Cookware of varying sizes: small and medium saucepot, skillet, high-sided skillet, large pot, Dutch oven (consider stainless steel or cast iron)
- Metal or bamboo steamer basket
- Baking sheet(s)
- Muffin tin(s)
- Cake pan(s)
- Parchment paper or Silpat liners
- Glass casserole dish
- French press or pour-over system
- Tea kettle
- *Optional: rice cooker, bread maker, wok, cast-iron skillet*

Prepping

- Wooden cutting boards
- Three to six fine knives that can be sharpened
- High-speed blender (like a Vitamix or Blendtec)
- Vegetable peeler
- Metal or glass mixing bowls
- Metal measuring cups
- Metal colander
- Metal tea diffuser (awesome for tea, but also great for infusing flavors into other liquids)

- Cheesecloth
- *Optional: spiralizer, salad* *spinner, tofu press, mandolin,*
  food processor, food scale

Dining

- Simple place settings/plates (if you fly solo, four large plates, four bowls, and four salad plates should be plenty)
- Glasses or repurposed jars for beverages
- Mugs (these are especially fun to get secondhand)
- Metal cutlery
- Serving utensils
- Cloth napkins (consider organic cotton, hemp, or linen)

Storage, Travel, Disposal, and Cleaning

- Mason jars with various lids for beverages and storage
- Glass or stainless-steel food storage options, with lids in varying sizes
- Silicone food-saver lids (awesome for popping on half-used cans or produce to prevent unnecessary spoilage)
- Silicone bags to replace plastic zip-type bags (I'm obsessed with these)
- Small metal containers with lids (for storing seeds and spices)
- Large glass carafes for water, iced tea, and large batches of boozy drinks
- Water-filtering pitcher, faucet attachment, or kishu charcoal for water filtration
- Stainless-steel bento boxes for packing lunches
- Bamboo or stainless-steel travel cutlery
- Reusable hot/cold bottle (for taking coffee or water to go)
- Cloth napkins
- Stainless-steel or glass straws
- Countertop composter
- Metal or wooden dish-drying rack
- Dish brush
- Cloth dish towels
- Castile soap for washing vegetables and dishes

NOT INTO LABELS

Some of the best containers for, well, everything are the jars, cans, and bottles from food, cleaning, and personal care items you've used. Spice shakers, glass jars and bottles, and aluminum cans are useful anywhere in the house, whether they're holding dry shampoo or a gerbera daisy. Instead of tossing these in the recycle bin, consider repurposing them as organizers, food storage, décor, and part of your waste-reducing on-the-go arsenal. But because faded spaghetti sauce stickers aren't considered HGTV chic, removing them is key to upcycling vessels to their utmost potential. Here's the truth: labels are a lot like exes—some are a cinch to get rid of, while others hang like Stacy in Wayne's World. For all of these I have a two-pronged approach that works wonders without fucking up your manicure.

* **Step 1: Soak:** After removing as much of the label as possible with your hands, submerge the item in hot water mixed with equal parts (about one tablespoon) white vinegar and castile soap. Let it soak for as long as you'd like to get things loose. Once soaked, use a dish brush or old toothbrush to rub away any remnants.

* **Step 2: Scrub:** If Step 1 hasn't sent your labels running, try a simple scrub. Dry off the item and mix one tablespoon of baking soda, one tea-spoon of vegetable oil, and a few drops of lemon essential oil together to form a thick, gritty paste. Either with a brush or your fingers, rub the mixture on the dry vessel to buff away hangers-on. The oils weaken the adhesive while the baking soda scrubs away the bits.

When shopping, look for products housed in reusable containers with limited labeling. Your nails will thank you.

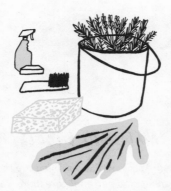

THE GIVE A SHIT
CLEANING KIT

Contrary to what marketers and advertisers would like us to think, unless you're running a crime scene hose-down biz, you don't need eight thousand products to come clean. Truly. But you will need a few things. And if you're looking at this list thinking, *Holy crap, that's a lot*, here I am to hold you close and whisper in your ear that many of these items (1) will do double (and sometimes triple) duty in your personal grooming and cooking arsenals and (2) can be handily and inexpensively upcycled from items you already have, like food containers, toothbrushes, and clothing fashioned into cleaning cloths. Bottom line: no need to get fancy or drop a lot of dough. Pick and choose what makes the most sense for you or blindly follow me like the lavender-infused cult leader I was born to be. YAS.

- Five upcycled glass bottles
- Two medium-sized Mason jars with lids
- Three upcycled soap pumps
- Two upcycled spray nozzles
- One to two metal or wooden scoops

- Two sustainable, reusable dual-sided sponges (one for the bathroom, one for the kitchen)
- Two sustainable (wire and wood) dish brushes—a smaller one for bottles, a larger one for everything else
- One upcycled (that is, used) toothbrush
- Dish-drying rack (even if you have a dishwasher, hand washing is efficient for smaller jobs and cuts down on sink pile-ups)
- Three-plus upcycled cloths for dusting, polishing, and throwing over your shoulder like you mean business
- One giant bottle of castile soap (whatever scent tickles your fancy, love)
- One bar of castile soap (I like tea tree)
- One large bottle of lemon essential oil
- One large bottle of tea tree essential oil
- Other essential oils you dig, like lavender, rose, rosemary, sandalwood
- One medium bottle of olive oil or other light vegetable oil (I prefer olive because it is easier to find in glass packaging)
- Baking soda
- White vinegar
- Borax
- Washing soda (which can also be made by heating baking soda; find instructions on page 93)
- Dryer balls (preferably vegan, nonwool versions)
- Rubber or upcycled gloves
- *Optional: French maid uniform*

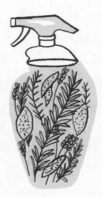

GREEN CLEANING RECIPES FOR YOUR ABODE

Making your own home cleaners may sound nauseatingly *Little House on the Prairie*, but I promise you're gonna dig it. These cleaners are easy on the environment, safe for your fam, and more affordable over time than the conventional crap, which are essentially just pricey cocktails of sickness-inducing chemicals and water swaddled in wasteful packaging.

Don't believe me? According to the EPA, a comprehensive test of conventional home cleaners on the shelves today showed that "each product emitted 1–8 toxic or hazardous chemicals, and close to half (44 percent) generated at least 1 of 24 carcinogenic hazardous air pollutants, such as acetaldehyde, 1,4-dioxane, formaldehyde, or methylene chloride. These hazardous air pollutants have no safe exposure level." That's bad news, friends. Seriously, although I need to issue the disclaimer that I am not a doctor, it doesn't take a rocket scientist to draw the conclusion that we shouldn't be slathering this stuff around our homes and all over our loved ones. Should you need further convincing, think about it this way: your kid or stoned roommate gets into the laundry room and downs a bottle of detergent (apparently this happens). What's the first thing you're supposed to do? If you answered "call Poison Control stat," you get a gold star (if not, don't babysit anyone ever—seriously). Why should you do this? Because that shit is POISON (and not in the cool Bell Biv DeVoe way). Conventional cleaners by law are not required to divulge all ingredients and can often contain the kinds of poisons that can wreck your insides.[52]

Creating cleaners is way easy, and you get to feel like a cool person whose home smells of citrus and smiles. Moreover, this shit really fucking works. If ever you come to my apartment, you'll understand the extent of my near-clinical tidiness and know that someone as filth averse as me would never proselytize the virtues of these concoctions unless they worked like the dickens. These DIY cleaners are:

- Nontoxic and healthier for all the living things in your home
- Cruelty-free
- Vegan
- Easy on waterways
- Low waste, with options to make zero waste
- More economical
- Smell, like, really, really nice
- Look cool and ultra-Instagrammable

INFUSED CLEANING VINEGAR

The not-so-secret operative in
all your squeaky-clean operations

You know how the father in *My Big Fat Greek Wedding* swears Windex is the cure-all for everything? Well, in this spinoff (My Big Fat Green Wedding?), that's how I feel about vinegar. It'll clean your home, hair, and mouth; keeps your gut healthy; and tastes great in a salad. It's also the cornerstone of most of the cleaning recipes in this here book. Why? Because it's cheap, safe, and works incredibly well. Because I'm a little extra, I like to spice mine up with some citrus and herbs I have hanging around. Citrus peels up the grease-cutting power and make the vinegar smell less vinegary. Aromatic herbs like lavender and rosemary are fun for adding aromatherapeutic benefits to the mix. Don't worry about perfection or precision here—feel free to explore combinations you like and keep it all in the fridge. If the solution begins to feel a bit lackluster, simply strain the additions from the vinegar, compost anything you no longer want in the infusion, and repeat the process!

INGREDIENTS

White vinegar

Citrus peels, saved from cooking

Lavender or rosemary sprigs, optional

TOOLS

Wide-mouthed glass jar and lid

Fill the jar two-thirds full with the vinegar. Add in your citrus peels and herbs of choice, if using. Cover with the lid, and store in the fridge for up to a month.

SPRAY SURFACE
CLEANER

*A grime-fighting superhero
in a reusable cloth cape*

The cabinet under my kitchen sink used to be a graveyard of spray bottles and various products purported to whip my home into pristine shape. Those have all been banished from the kingdom since I started using this magically simple cleaner. Bathroom mirrors? Streak-free! Grimy counters and surfaces? Sparklin'! And the best part? If you're running low, you can simply add to your current batch bottle and keep that spray going.

INGREDIENTS

2 tablespoons of that kickass Infused Cleaning Vinegar (opposite)
you're keeping in your fridge, or plain white vinegar

2 teaspoons liquid castile soap
(I like Dr. Bronner's Sal Suds)

2 cups water, or however much is needed to fill your bottle

5–10 drops essential oils such as tea tree,
lavender, or lemon

TOOLS

Repurposed spray cleaner bottle with nozzle,
or glass bottle and a repurposed spray nozzle (you'll be surprised
how easily a lot of these fit other bottles—I use a repurposed
apple cider vinegar glass bottle fitted with the spray nozzle from
one of those aforementioned graveyard bottles
and I'm in business)

Combine the vinegar, castile soap, and water in your container, then add your desired essential oils; feel free to experiment with different ratios and scent combinations (I like to mix 4 drops each of tea tree and lavender or just do a full 10 drops of lemon). Shake it up, spray it 'round! Easy peasy.

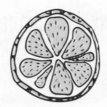

SIMPLE CITRUS SCRUB

Would make the bathtub from Silence of the Lambs
smell like a lemon grove

As a child, I had chores. Remember those? One of my chores was to clean the bathtub, and let me tell you, I fucking hated it. I'd rather pull weeds for hours in the oppressive Texas summer sun, emerging dirty, lobster red, and covered in mosquito bites, than scrub filthy grout (and often times I'd beg to do just that, with the conviction of a *Hunger Games* tribute). So, Soft Scrub and sponge in hand, off I'd trudge to the bathroom after much prodding from my parents. One time, when I was eight years old, I spent the entire day sitting on the bathroom floor perusing a *Reader's Digest* with the water running just to give my parents the illusion that I was really giving it my all. Imagine their surprise when, four hours later, the bathroom was no different, but I'd acquired a near-encyclopedic knowledge of the cast of *227*. #grounded.

That said, as one becomes an adult, such things need to get done because no matter how great your bosom, no one wants to make out with you when your bathroom looks like a set out of *C.S.I.* Plus, nowadays, cleaning isn't so bad. Why? Probably because this simple scrub smells hella good and works like magic. And it's not just for showers: I use this beauty to get metal and porcelain of all types (tea kettles, old baking pans, stovetops, knife blades, even certain jewelry) sparkling—everything *including* the (metal) kitchen sink. It's also excellent for removing sticky labels from jars and cans. Best of all, it's totally cruelty-free and assimilates safely into waterways (no pollution or creepy microbeads!) while still being effective as hell and making everything smell lemony fresh.

INGREDIENTS

2 cups baking soda

25–30 drops lemon essential oil (*Not* lemon juice.
Don't cut corners here, guys. And buy the largest size you can get—
it will last you a long time, and you'll use it for everything.)

TOOLS

Sustainable dual-sided sponge or
wooden scrub brush

Repurposed used toothbrush

The process may sound tedious, but it's kind of like watching magic happen before your very eyes, and magic is always worth the effort. Pour some baking soda on a wet, wrung-out sponge or brush. Then add a few drops of lemon essential oil atop the baking soda. Now, apply that fucker to the semidry surface of whatever you're trying to clean, and get to scrubbin'. The dry grit of the baking soda combined with the grease-eradicating power of the essential oil make for a beautiful result. Once you've thoroughly scrubbed, rinse the surface well and marvel at what a badass housekeeper you've become. If you're cleaning grout or little crannies, dip the toothbrush into the baking soda, add a few drops of oil, and go to town. Okay, I'll leave you to it.

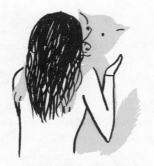

LAVENDER–TEA TREE DETERGENT

So fresh and so clean, clean

Much as I disliked bathroom duty, I've blossomed into one of those weirdos who finds laundry oddly therapeutic. I put this detergent to the test when I adopted my pup, Banjo. She'd murder me for telling this story (sorry, B), but it really drives home how effective this recipe is at handling even the biggest laundry S.O.S. ever. (Trigger warning: if you're eating, stop reading now.) After visiting Banjo, then named Shayla, at the shelter for about three weeks, I made our nonsexual life partnership official on a rainy Sunday afternoon. Like all good first dates, we were both excited, a little nervous, and kinda relieved—I because she was safe and sound, and she because shelters can be stressful places. She was so relieved, in fact, that she sashayed into my apartment, made a cozy spot for herself on my bed, and then proceeded to SHIT ALL OVER said bed. I'm talkin' pillows, blankets, the afghan my grand-mother knitted—the works. I understood: she was comfortable and finally felt safe. I also couldn't stop gagging. Fast forward: this detergent and hot water saved my linens, the day, and our relationship. So whether you've got run-of-the-mill laundry or a holy-shit-help-me-Jesus bodily fluids situation, this—and maybe a gas mask—is all you need.

This detergent is highly effective at removing stains, brightening whites, and making clothes smell fresh in a clean, unisex way. And yes, it's safe for front-loading and high-efficiency machines as well as effective for hand washing. Sometimes I just use liquid castile soap as my detergent, and that's lovely, especially when I'm hand washing. But when I want something with a bit more oomph and stain-removing power, this is my go-to recipe. (I also cover below how to make your own washing soda to use in the detergent; many folks do not wish to use store-bought washing soda because some brands test on animals, and to that I say, *you go, Glen Coco*.)

FOR THE HOMEMADE WASHING SODA

INGREDIENTS

2 cups baking soda

Tools

Glass casserole dish

FOR THE DETERGENT

INGREDIENTS

1 cup Homemade Washing Soda

1 cup Borax

1 bar tea tree castile soap

20-plus drops lavender essential oil

10-plus drops tea tree essential oil

TOOLS

Cheese grater or sharp knife

High-powered blender

Wide-mouthed jar and lid

Metal or wooden scoop

First, make the washing soda: Crank your oven to 400°F, put a ½-inch-thick layer of baking soda in a casserole dish, and let that soda bake for 1 to 1½ hours, stirring occasionally. You'll know you've gone from bakin' to washin' when the texture becomes grainier. Chemistry! Science! Oh, the wonder! You'll also have a bit more than you need for this detergent recipe, so simply store the extra in a glass jar and it'll be ready when you need to make more detergent.

Now, for the detergent: Use the grater or a sharp knife to break down the bar soap for easier grinding. Place all the ingredients in the dry container of a high-powered blender, like a Vitamix, and pulse until you have a fine powder (this may take a minute and that's ok). Add more essential oil as needed, blend again, then store in a glass jar with a scoop.

Use 2 tablespoons per medium-sized load of laundry, or as needed for hand washing and soaking. I like to add it to the water and once it's diluted a bit, add my clothes.

QUICK HITS
IN YOUR HOME

There are oh-so-many ways to make positive changes in your home, but these are a few that will totally rock your socks in a short amount of time.

- *Research recycling in your area. Make a plan to stick with the program and start recycling right.*

- *FOR THE LOVE OF ALL THAT'S HOLY: Vow to stop buying single-use beverage containers, like plastic water bottles, right freaking now.*

- *Following the steps on page 56, put yourself (and an elderly relative or neighbor, if you have time) on as many unsubscribe lists as possible to cut down on the barrage of junk mail making your foyer impassible.*

- *When not in use, turn off the fucking faucet, television, and lights. You're grown. You can do this.*

- *Skip the dishwasher and give your daily dishes some hands-on attention.*

- *Wash small clothing items like socks and undies by hand, or save them up for a machine wash when you've got a truly full load.*

- *Swap paper towels for reusable, washable cloths. That's it. World saved.*

- *Inherit, rescue (from Craigslist), or invest in one of the air-cleaning plants listed on page 50.*

- *If you're able, turn your water heater temp down to 120°F.*

- *Look around your home. Do you have a lot of stuff you don't really use? If so, make a plan to downsize, and when you legitimately need an item, consider resource sharing or getting it secondhand.*

Give a Shit:

In the Kitchen

I'd be remiss if I wrote a book on sustainable living and didn't cover the most impactful action you can take to save the planet—eat fewer (or, better yet, no) animal products. Now, before you go all Hulk on me and rip this book in half with the fury of a thousand cookouts, I'm not here to preach or judge. It has, however, been scientifically proven that animal agriculture is seriously killing the planet. Well-respected entities like the United Nations and thoroughly researched, longitudinal studies have found that animal agriculture, even of the often-applauded "sustainable" or "humane" ilks, packs more of a negative wallop to our planet than all transportation industries combined.[1] All. Transportation. Industries. Combined. WTF, right? Every plane, train, automobile, ship, and cat in a shark costume riding a Roomba (maybe not that last one . . .) in the world combined erode less of the ozone and use fewer resources than the seemingly innocuous steak on your plate. Normally I'd be open to critical discourse on this, but really, this is fucking science, guys. The planet is becoming a shit show, and it's largely because of how we eat.

Recycling, buying secondhand, composting, turning off the lights—these are all awesome steps toward lessening your carbon footprint. But if you're type A like me and want to effect the most positive change with a singular step, it's time to get comfy with plant-powered grub. Luckily this "holy crap I'm saving the world" step is pretty damn easy and enjoyable, and how often does that happen? The average American eats an astounding 209 pounds of meat per year, and you can make a dent in that digit every time you pick up your fork.[2] Other purported bonuses of a plant-strong dietary shift include smaller grocery bills, a healthier waistline, and increased energy, mood, and libido, to name a few. Don't take it from me, though. Doctors are already on top of this stuff, and from what I've heard, some of those peeps really know their shit.

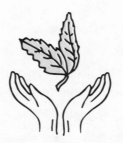

FIND YOUR REASON
FOR VEGAN

As with any new habit (like working out or showing up to meetings on time), in order for it to stick, you need to find your reason. The nice part about plant-based eating is that there's no single benefit or impetus—there are oh-so many. Whether you're passionate about the environment (which, I'm guessing you are because you're reading this book), social justice, good health, or good karma, there's a compelling rationale for curbing your intake. Some folks stumble into a plant-based diet for health reasons. Others, like myself, have an epiphany after their shelter dog stares at them for two solid hours and they realize they want to live in a way that's more aligned with the values of protecting vulnerable creatures. And hell, I've even met a few people who are just cheap as fuck and want the most nutrient density for their buck in the form of bulk beans, legumes, grains, and vegetables.

Here's the thing: once you start eating in a more vegan way, people are going to become weirdly obsessed with your lifestyle, nutrient intake, and probably even your digestion. So in addition to laying out the multitudinous reasons plant-based eating is a huge step in the right direction, feel free to use the following as slaying talking points when overserved Uncle Jeff tries to convince everyone that you're a pansy because you won't eat the Easter ham.

Climate Change

Although the methodologies and results vary, loads of research bodies, from the University of Oxford to the United Nations, have cited animal agriculture as being responsible for anywhere between 14.5 percent to a staggering 51 percent of greenhouse gas emissions.[3] That's more than the exhaust from all modes of transportation in the world combined. Now if you're about to protest that not all farming operations are large scale or industrialized enough to make a dent, it's important to remember that nearly 99 percent of all farm animals in the United States are raised on one of the eighteen thousand–plus American factory farms, also known as concentrated animal feeding operations (CAFOs).[4]

As anyone who's ever fed their dog popcorn knows, animals can be gassy bastards. Factory-farmed animals, especially the 102 million flatulent cattle and calves reported in 2017, account for more than 9 percent of global carbon dioxide, 35 to 40 percent of global methane, and 65 percent of nitrous oxide emissions.[5] Methane is especially insidious because it can trap one hundred times more heat in the atmosphere than CO_2, which, as you might gather, really warms ye olde climate.[6] But toots aren't the only things that make CAFOs such planet destroyers. Like the uninvited moocher who drinks all of your home brew, animal agriculture uses more than a third of all fossil fuels consumed in the United States.[7,8] And this is just the appetizer, kids.

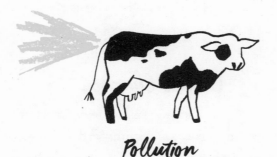

Pollution

Animals are living things, and living things produce waste. It's sort of part of the whole "existing" deal. And that waste pollutes waterways, soil, air, and nearby communities because, well, the shit's gotta go somewhere. Every second in the United States, animals raised for food produce 116,000 pounds of excrement, and that stat doesn't include the billions of fish raised in aquaculture settings.[9] In America, 130 times more animal waste than human waste is produced, which is enough to cover San Francisco, New York

City, Tokyo, and a bunch of other cities that are too expensive for me to live in.[10] To think of this more manageably, a modest dairy of 2,500 cows can produce the same amount of waste as a city of 411,000 people.[11]

Unlike human excrement, however, factory-farm waste is not processed as sewage, largely because, as evidenced above, there's simply way too fucking much of it. Because it's left untreated, this waste is five hundred times more concentrated than human waste and is rife with intact pathogens (like salmonella and *E. coli*), antibiotics, and volatile chemicals.[12] So what do many CAFOs do with all this toxic crap? Well, first some see how much can be absorbed in soil neighboring the CAFO. Once that's exhausted, some manure is used as fertilizer, spraying it into the air and on crops with a giant shit hose (isn't that a fun mental picture?).[13] Both scenarios introduce an overabundance of phosphorous and nitrogen into water systems, thereby causing ecosystem-choking algae blooms that, to date, are estimated to have impaired 170,750 miles of US rivers.[14]

After that literal shit show, remaining waste (of which there is still A LOT) festers in open-air, multimillion-gallon cesspools sneakily called lagoons.[15] Doesn't that sound cool? I mean, who wouldn't want to live near a giant pool of poo?! What could go wrong? Well, in addition to wafting stench to neighboring communities, these turd lagoons emit hundreds of harmful gasses like nitrous oxide, hydrogen sulfide, and ammonia that can sicken nearby residents with respiratory issues like asthma, seizures, poor mental health, and a host of other health problems.[16] To sweeten the deal, because 80 percent of antibiotics sold in the United States are given to farm animals, those agents like tetracycline can contaminate the air, water, and ground, creating problematic overexposure for and possible bacterial resistance in humans.[17]

Habitat Destruction
and Extinction

Although the earth is freaking huge, habitable space is not in endless supply. Livestock and their feed occupy one-third of the planet's habitable (as in, not a giant block of ice) land and 45 percent of the planet's total land, with an estimated two to five acres of land used per cow.[18] Domestically, half of the contiguous United States is devoted to animal agriculture.[19] HALF. Oh, and have you ever heard of this pretty important thing called the Amazon rainforest? Well, animal agriculture—namely livestock and associated feed crops—is estimated to be responsible for up to 91 percent of its destruction.[20]

Demand for cheap, readily available meat requires more grazing room, to the tune of 136 million rainforest acres cleared each year, 80 percent of which is used for cattle pasture.[21] This sucks for many reasons.[22] Once believed to be a "carbon sink," the Amazon absorbed more carbon than it produced (that's a good thing). However, current deforestation and other activities have significantly reduced its absorption to about even with the region's emissions (that's not a good thing).[23] Being the most biodiverse space on the planet, 137 plant, animal, and insect species—all of whom are incredibly vital to our delicate ecosystem—are lost every freaking day due to Amazon destruction. Indigenous peoples, including uncontacted tribes of hunter-gatherers (believed to be perhaps the oldest human societies—no biggie), can not only lose their homes and culture but can often fall victim to enslavement and exploitation.[24]

Oh, and remember when we talked about those gassy animals awhile back? Well, all that ammonia emitted from their excrement combines with other pollutants to form nitric acid, which returns

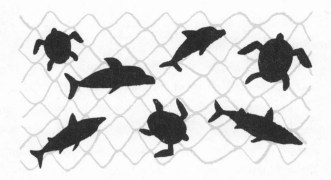

ROUGH SEAS

And let's talk about oceans for a sec. I'm a fan. But horrible things are happening to our oceans because of our consumption habits. Although the amount of sea life we directly kill for food each year in the United States is unknown, estimates can reach into twenty-two billion–plus, and numbers often don't include sport and recreational fishing.[i] And those are just the sea creatures that are the "desired catch." Most fishing methods, like trawlers, which are giant nets that scrape up everything in their paths, catch and kill thousands of unintended animals, deemed "bycatch." Remember when "Dolphin Safe" tuna was all the rage? That's because the public caught wind of dolphins suffering due to commercial tuna fishing methods—but bycatch happens in almost every commercial fishing scenario. Scientists estimate as many as 650,000 whales, dolphins, and seals are killed each year by fishing vessels and that forty to fifty million sharks are killed in fishing lines and nets annually.[ii] These animals are critical to upholding the delicate symbiosis of the ocean and our planet's ecosystem as a whole.

Let me break this down on an individual level: For every American's annual seafood intake, it's estimated that up to 104 unintended creatures—like seals, turtles, sharks, dolphins, smaller crustaceans, and more—are captured, killed, or discarded.[iii] And due to these detrimental blanket commercial fishing methods, overfishing to meet our rampant demand, pollution, habitat destruction, and rapidly heating and acidic ocean conditions, marine populations are no longer able to replenish themselves at their natural rates, often to the point of endangerment and extinction. If our consumption and commercialization don't straighten up and swim right, the UN has estimated that we could see entirely fishless oceans by 2050.[iv] That shrimp cocktail doesn't seem quite as appetizing anymore, huh?

to the earth's surface as acid rain, which is also terrible for forests, oceans, and, well, everything.[25]

At home the USDA's Wildlife Services branch conducts mass exterminations (which they refer to as "culls") of wild animals, sometimes in the name of protecting livestock raised for food. And protecting livestock means various things, like ensuring grazing land isn't trolled by other animals, under the clauses allowing this horror show, which is funded by your taxpayer dollars. In 2016 the USDA reported killing 76,963 adult coyotes, 21,184 beavers, 14,654 prairie dogs, 3,791 foxes, 997 bobcats, 415 gray wolves, 407 black bears, 334 mountain lions, and 535 river otters.[26] Although it's all a bit more hush-hush, the Department of Interior's Bureau of Land Management (BLM) has engaged in similar roundups of wild horses and burros. Because rehoming horses is expensive and populations are booming, the bureau is allowed to sell certain animals to slaughter and, in 2017, asked that restrictions on "the sale and disposition of excess animals" be lifted.[27] The biggest cheerleader for these culls: the National Cattlemen's Beef Association. Why? Wild mustangs encroach on terrain needed for livestock.[28] I'm not trying to be Pollyanna here: overpopulation happens and brings with it difficult ecosystemic dilemmas. However, it seems logical to assume that the fewer CAFOs, and the lessened demand for meat, the more habitat for these wild and vital creatures to thrive.

Resource Consumption

Animal agriculture is responsible for 20 to 33 percent of global freshwater consumption today, which is pretty nutty when we consider that 10 percent of the world's population doesn't have reliable access to potable water.[29] Animals require resources, and large numbers of animals require—you guessed it—large amounts of resources. Worldwide, it's estimated cows drink 45 billion gallons of water and eat 135 billion pounds of food each day.[30] In America 55 percent of water, 70 percent of grain, and 33 percent of fossil fuels are used for farmed animals.[31] To put this in an on-your-plate perspective, one pound of beef guzzles anywhere from 442 to 2,500 gallons of water, and a gallon of milk chugs 1,000 gallons. If you're saying, "Well, plants require resources too," I say, "Of course," but please chew on this: it takes about twelve times as much land, thirteen times as much fossil fuel, and fifteen times as much water to produce a pound of animal protein as it does a pound of soy protein.[32] Although all food products have some associated resource consumption, animal products rank notoriously high.

Resource Inequity and Privilege

In the Introduction I touched on how data shows that climate change will adversely impact poorer, low-lying countries first. Animal agriculture also presents similar issues when it comes to global resources. Chief among them: how is it ethical to feed thousands of pounds of life-sustaining grain to fatten a cow when 14 million people are starving in Yemen?[33] Here's the sitch: 11.3 percent of the world's population is hungry. That's roughly 805 million people who go undernourished on a daily basis.[34] And it's not because we don't produce enough food to feed all 7.5 billion people on the planet (we actually produce enough food to feed 10 billion. Call us overachievers), but rather because those who go hungry either do not have land or money to grow or purchase food, or the food they can purchase is in shorter supply because it's used to feed and fatten animals.[35] Don't buy it? Half of all the world's grain is used to feed livestock, and 82 percent of starving children live in countries where the grain grown is fed to animals, and those animals are in turn largely consumed by and in Western countries.[36] That, my friends, is not only bullshit; it is the essence of gratuitous privilege, and when we give a shit, we don't play that way.

Animal Suffering

File this one under DUH: animals suffer greatly in our industrialized food system.[37] Yes, even the "humanely raised," Kosher, cage-free, Halal, free-range, #blessed (or whatever nouveau, feel-good murder term the kids are using these days) ones can suffer. Don't let such terms impart a false sense of comfort. Under the Humane Methods of Slaughter Act, "humane" simply necessitates that animals—except for chickens and turkeys, who are woefully omitted from the language—be stunned at the time of slaughter (not very comforting).[38] However, the fast-paced, profit-driven nature of conventional animal agriculture and the sheer volume of incoming animals (an estimated ten billion land animals—we're not even talking fish here—every year in the United States alone[39]) mean that proper stunning isn't always achieved. Moreover, because efficiency is king in any kind of processing, it's been purported that some processors believe that the fastest way to drain animals of blood is to slit their throats while their hearts are still beating.[40] Put the last two sentences together and what do you get? A whole hell of a lot of sentient creatures potentially suffering because they're literally bleeding out while still conscious.

I hate to bust up a Santa Claus–level myth for you guys, but at no point ever has an animal gone to the farmer, offered her neck, and said, "Farmer Bill, it's time." And if you're going to eat meat and animal products, the least you can do is be woke about how these creatures live and eventually die. I'm going to give you the realities some of these animals face as unemotionally as possible—in the form of an HR-style chart. Now, this chart outlines what *can* happen in *some* traditional, large-scale animal agriculture situations. While animal-lovers-cum-realists like myself tend to believe this shit happens on a much wider scale (not to mention the whole "animals aren't consenting to these fates" thing), I do want to add the don't-sue-me-because-I'm-broke caveat that this is not *every* CAFO's process or *every* animal's experience. This is a day-to-day explanation of what the laws (at the time of penning this book) allow for large-scale, conventional animal rearing and processing in the United States. So if you feel shook reading this, I'd say that's your conscience kicking in and, as Mom said, listen to that little voice.

FROM FRIENDS TO FOOD: HOW SOME ANIMALS LIVE AND DIE IN TRADITIONAL LARGE-SCALE AGRICULTURE [41]

COMMODITY	ANIMAL	HOW SOME LIVE	HOW SOME DIE
Pork	Pigs	Tails are docked, ends of teeth are removed with pliers, and male piglets are castrated often without pain relief. Mother sows can be kept in gestation and farrowing crates so small they cannot turn around. Male hogs are often confined and crowded. Mother sows are often forcibly inseminated, and their piglets are removed a few weeks after birth. Spent sows, male pigs, and suckling piglets are transported on cramped trucks. Depending on the season, it is estimated that one million pigs die in transit each year from causes such as heat exhaustion, disease, lameness, or freezing to death.	Immobilization renders some pigs too weak to walk. Others, excited to experience space for the first time, begin to run for the first time in their lives. Forced through a chute and then stunned via an electric current, captive bolt pistol, or inhalation of CO_2. In some cases a .22 pistol/rifle is shot directly into the brain. Hoisted on a rail and exsanguinated through carotid artery or jugular vein. Once bled out, some pigs are dragged through boiling water via a pig scalder to remove hair. Hair is further removed using scissor-devices or torches. As a typical slaughterhouse kills eleven hundred pigs per hour, it is possible that some animals can be improperly stunned and thus, remain conscious through many or all of the above processes.
Chicken Poultry	Chickens	Beaks and sometimes toes, spurs, and combs are cut off using a hot blade often with no pain relief. Broiler chickens (bred for meat) can be crowded and confined in windowless sheds with thousands of other birds and sent to slaughter around six to seven weeks of age. Breeder chickens (birthing hens) can be similarly crowded and confined but are not sent to slaughter until their breeding use is exhausted. Due to husbandry, like selective breeding to create larger, faster-growing birds, and drugs catalyzing unnatural rapid growth, some chickens suffer heart attacks, organ failure, and crippling deformities that prevent them from accessing water nozzles. Transported to slaughter in packed trucks.	Due to rough handling during transport, some chickens arrive to slaughter with broken wings and legs. Their legs are often shackled, throats are slit, and bodies are dredged through scalding defeathering tanks. Since stunning is not legally required for chickens, it is possible that some animals experience the above while still conscious.

Illustrations © GettyImages/Kittisak_Taramas

Turkey Poultry	Turkeys	Often genetically bred to grow as quickly as possible, turkeys can experience lameness and immobilization due to excess weight.	Hung upside down by their legs and dragged through an electrified stunning tank that immobilizes but does not kill them.
		Toes, upper beaks, and snoods are often removed with a hot blade and no pain relief.	Due to volume and struggle of animals, it's possible for birds to miss the tank so they can sometimes be completely conscious as their throats are slit.
		Can be packed into dark sheds with no more than three and a half square feet of space per bird.	
		Sent to slaughter at five to six months old, despite a natural lifespan of ten years.	Struggle can also result in imprecise throat-slitting, so some animals can be conscious and scalded to death in boiling water used for defeathering.
		Slaughter transport is sometimes their first opportunity to feel the sun or wind. Up to two thousand turkeys can be crammed into transport trucks without food or water for up to 28 hours and are exposed to harsh elements.	
Beef	Cattle	Dehorned, castrated, and branded often without painkillers.	Often forced through a chute and shot in the head with a captive-bolt gun.
		Fattened on feedlots where they can endure harsh temperatures, crowding, waste, and disease.	Throats are slit, and animals are dismembered. As stunning can be imprecise, some animals may endure the above while still conscious and without pain relief.
		Transported long distances in packed trucks where they can receive no food, water, or breaks, and can languish in waste and downed animals for up to twenty-eight hours.	
Veal	Calves	Usually separated from their mothers immediately upon or up to three days after birth. Trauma from removal and lack of access to mother's milk can result in visible distress and disease.	Some calves arrive to slaughter unable to walk due to immobilization and severe underdevelopment.
		Shipped to feedlots to await slaughter or placed in hutches, crates, (typically two and a half feet wide) or small group pens. Confines can be intentionally small to restrict movement and preserve tenderness of meat.	If they are able to rise and walk from a recumbent position after showing signs of lameness, they can be slaughtered similarly to other cows.
		Intentionally fed a liquid diet, sometimes devoid of iron and fiber (which can result in anemia) to create a "creamy white to pale pink" flesh often deemed more desirable by consumers.	
		Typically slaughtered around sixteen to twenty weeks of age. About fifteen percent of veal calves, called bobs, are slaughtered at three weeks old for lower-grade products.	

| Seafood Fish | Fish, lobsters, crabs | Half of all fish consumed are raised on land- or ocean-based aquafarms confined by net enclosures.

Crowding can encourage parasitic infections, diseases, and injuries.

Can be starved for up to ten days prior to slaughter to avoid waste contamination during transport.

Non-aquacultured sea life can be commercially fished using long lines (often fifty-plus miles of baited hooks), weighted gill nets (often three hundred feet to seven miles long), purse seines (which can unintentionally trap and kill dolphins), bottom trawlers (bag-shaped nets pulled along the ocean floor by boat), shallow water traps (more commonly used for crabs and lobsters), and more traditional pole and line methods. | Without any legal protection, fish can be impaled, crushed, suffocated, frozen, boiled, or gutted while fully conscious.

Commercial fishing also results in the death of nontarget or bycatch animals, including sharks, sea turtles, birds, seals, dolphins, and whales. |
| Dairy | Cows | Often forcibly inseminated each year.

Can spend most of their lives pregnant and standing up in waste, which can render some (certain studies estimate up to about 50 percent) lame at the end of their lives.

Can be bred to have unnatural reproductive capacity and given growth hormones that can cause painfully inflamed udders (mastitis).

Calves are often removed from their mother within a day of birth, which can cause extreme maternal distress. Female calves are prepped for dairy life, while male calves are prepped to become veal.

After separation, a mother cow can be hooked up to a milking machine that could extract up to one hundred pounds of her milk a day.

The cycle repeats until cows become spent (around five years, despite a natural lifespan of twenty years).

Transported long distances in packed trucks with conditions similar to those experienced by cattle en route to slaughter. | Some dairy cows arrive to slaughter "downed," or too lame or sick to walk or stand.

Able-bodied cows are forced through a chute and can be shot in the head with a captive-bolt gun.

Downed cows are illegal to process, but some footage and accounts have shown downed animals being pushed to slaughter with bulldozers.

Throats are slit, and animals are dismembered. Given the possibility for error in stunning, some animals experience the above while still conscious and without pain relief. |

Eggs	Chickens	From birth to 10 days old, many hens' beaks are removed with an infrared blade often without pain relief.	Hen slaughter is similar to that of broiler and breeding chickens, and no stunning is required by law.
		At 16 weeks of age, some birds are placed in battery cages (illegal in certain states) with other birds, experiencing only 67 to 86 square inches of space each, or about the size of an A4 sheet of paper. Such confinement often means that birds cannot move their wings and can stand in feces and downed animals.	Male baby chicks, worthless to the egg industry, are macerated in high-speed grinders while still alive or suffocated to death with no anesthesia upon hatching.
		Light and feed levels are manipulated to maximize and induce egg laying.	
		Upon being classified as spent (around two years of age), hens are transported to slaughter.	

Worker Exploitation and Suffering

As is the case with workers in general agriculture, the estimated five hundred thousand slaughterhouse and meat processing workers in America are predominantly lower-income persons of color, 38 percent of whom were born outside of the United States, with an unknown but anecdotally assumed large percentage being undocumented.[42] Poor working conditions and barely livable wages ($11.21 an hour in 2012) mean that astronomically high turnover (250 percent in some cases) is an industry norm. Among undocumented workers, who receive little to no labor and legal protections, the threat of deportation is often unfairly used as coercion to toil longer hours for little money and few benefits.[43]

The nature of animal "processing" (air quotes because you just read the chart above and "processing" is way too bizarre a word for that shit show) is fast paced—fueled by consumer demand for cheap meat—and arduous with sharp, heavy equipment; oppressive temperatures; frantic, flailing animals (remember the scene from *Tommy Boy* where the deer is in the back of the car? That. All day.); chemicals; and emitted gasses and waste that present significant safety hazards. It's been deemed one of the most dangerous jobs, with three times the injury risk rate of that of an average American factory and a reported 25 percent of slaughterhouse workers becoming ill on the job.[44]

And as awful as that all sounds, the physical wounds of animal processing pale in comparison to the emotional and mental fuckery. I mean, think about it: you roll up to your first day at a new job, and your boss is like, "Welcome aboard! Today I need you to electrocute one thousand freaked pigs fighting for their lives." Fuuuuuuck. Although it's true that most Americans are deeply disconnected from the animals they eat, the slaughterhouse is a point of acute, inescapable connectivity. Studies show slaughterhouse workers have high incidences of perpetration-induced traumatic stress (PITS), a form of posttraumatic stress disorder with symptoms of drug and alcohol abuse, panic, depression, paranoia, dissociation, and anxiety stemming from the act of killing.[45] A former kill floor manager (yes, that's a real job title) gave the following account:

> The worst thing—worse than the physical danger—is the emotional toll. . . . Pigs down on the kill floor have come up and nuzzled me like a puppy. Two minutes later I had to kill them— beat them to death with a pipe. I can't care.[46]

Moreover, this desensitization to killing can cross over from animals to people. Case in point: a 2010 study found a strong correlation (a 130 percent increase in some areas) between the presence of large slaughterhouses and high violent-crime rates, like child abuse, in US communities.[47] Workers responsible for initially terminating an animal, like "stickers," who literally stab hogs to death with sharp metal rods, are believed to be more susceptible:

> When I worked upstairs taking hogs' guts out, I could cop an attitude that I was working on a production line, helping to feed people. But down in the stick pit, I wasn't feeding people. I was killing things. My attitude was, it's only an animal. Kill it. Sometimes I looked at people that way, too. I've had ideas of hanging my foreman upside down on the line and sticking him. I remember going into the office and telling the personnel man that I have no problem pulling the trigger on a person— if you get in my face, I'll blow you away. Every sticker I know carries a gun, and every one of them would shoot you. Most stickers I know have been arrested for assault.[48]

I'm not crying; you're crying (wait, we're all crying because this is incredibly freaking sad). And if you're thinking to yourself, *Why don't they just get a different job?*, I gather you've probably never been a destitute or desperate refugee or poor at all. Newsflash: it's fucking difficult out there for the little guy, and some animal ag head honchos prey on the vulnerable, both people and animals, to turn a profit. Let me leave ya with this final point: when asked, 85 percent of carnivores surveyed said they'd be unwilling to kill the meat they eat.[49] So why would we expect others to do it for us if we know they suffer greatly in the process?

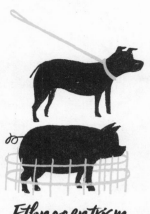

Ethnocentrism

Have you heard of the Yulin Dog Meat Festival? If not, it's a large celebration in China where they wrangle street dogs and eat them. Yes, I find it disturbing. But no more disturbing than the nonfestive daily ritual of American animal slaughter. I bring this up to illustrate ethnocentrism, which is basically a fancy term for cultural racism, because really, what's the difference between a dog and a cow, aside from the fact that we Western folk have decided that dogs are domesticated creatures worthy of protection and cows are agricultural commodities? If you've ever met a cow, you'd know they're so much like puppies, it's ridiculous—they frolic, snuggle, and have such sweet, long eyelashes. And most importantly, they have the same scientifically proven ability to feel pain, fear, and love as dogs or any other mammals do. Ancient Romans ate flamingoes, jungle-dwelling Bolivians eat monkeys and insects, and in France horse meat is considered a delicacy. The point here is that since when were Westerners granted dominion over which animals are and are not worthy of protection? And moreover, who are we to say that one culture is whack because their rubric is different from ours? That's basically the essence of cultural racism, and although it's certainly not a phenomenon limited to what we eat, we give a shit and are better than that.

Poor Health

According to the Academy of Nutrition and Dietetics, plant-strong peeps are less likely to develop heart disease, cancer, diabetes, or high blood pressure. Studies also show that vegetarians are on average ten-plus pounds lighter and live three to six years longer than their carnivorous counterparts.[50] Americans consume twice as much protein as necessary for a healthy diet, most of which is from red meat, and fifteen million Americans take prescription statins to reduce cholesterol.[51] Do you know what can only be found in animal products? Cholesterol! So it's pretty logical to conclude that eating less meat and more plants can help to ease the epidemic of cholesterol-influenced cardiovascular conditions and fatalities. Plant-based diets have also been linked to improvement in breath, body odor, skin, allergies, PMS, migraines, mood, energy, and libido.[52]

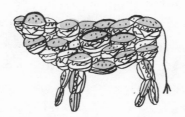

Cognitive Dissonance

If you're someone who leans a little *X Files*, you'll really like this one. Why? Because the truth is out there and it will set you free. The success of the Westernized food system relies heavily on consumers' cognitive dissonance. For one, the animal products we buy at the store are so removed from any association with the creatures from which they came. Chickens are plucked and fashioned into panko-crusted nuggets, pigs are ground into tidy little sausages, and cows are formed into round patties. Not a day goes by on social media when you don't see a story of someone wigging out because they found a vein or webbed foot in their bucket of fried chicken. No shit, person—what you're eating came from a living creature with veins and feet. If we're real with ourselves, a chicken wing or breast is one of two essential appendages on a single chicken. Veal is a dairy industry byproduct, a male calf who can't produce milk, so we eat his baby body because "it's soooooo tender!" Dairy products are postnatal milk stolen from a mother cow who spends her entire life pregnant via forced insemination (which, when done to a person sans consent, is rape), standing up, and having her babies taken from her. Eggs are poultry periods, usually begot from chickens crammed so tightly together that the human equivalent would be us spending our lives in a shit-infested elevator packed with twelve completely deranged people who eventually try to eat each other. I know: it's sad and grody. It's also by design.

This smoke-and-mirrors approach of American animal agriculture isn't limited to product packaging, display, and marketing either. Ever taken a cross-country road trip? Most slaughterhouse transport trucks make their journeys at night partly because they know even the most ardent carnivores find the sight of thousands of frantic pigs crammed in a perforated metal container on their way to a nasty fate to be—you guessed it—fucking distressing.[53] Feedlots and slaughterhouses are often located in more remote, less densely populated areas because, as Sir Paul McCartney said, "If slaughterhouses had glass walls, everyone would be a vegetarian." And he's a Beatle, guys.

There's a highly orchestrated system that makes this cognitive dissonance such an easy trap. We grow up with a USDA-approved food pyramid espousing meat and dairy as "essential food groups," and national holidays like Thanksgiving that literally revolve around animal sacrifice. If you're entrenched in eating animal products, don't beat yourself up—you've been habituated to believe that carnism is not only normal but essential. The good news is that with information and activism, you can easily free yourself from the status quo. And if you have your doubts, just remember that things like slavery, women not being allowed to hold jobs, and bedazzled jeans were once widely accepted as societal norms. Let's evolve, shall we?

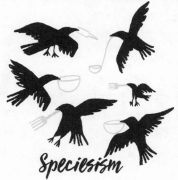

Speciesism

It's as if people having opposable thumbs is akin to the kind of hubris that a dude with a large penis or a sports car develops. Yeah, people are cool and all, but are we really the apex of existence and skill? One trip to a big-box store on a weekend will have you screaming into the void, "I HOPE NOT!" Allow me to brag on some holy-shit-worthy animal capabilities:

→ Octopuses can learn to open child protective caps (let's be real, most people can't ace that shit). Oh, and they can execute cognitive tasks even when dismembered.[54]

→ Dogs and other domesticated animals like horses can pick up on nonverbal, physical human cues. A skill your close-talker coworker clearly hasn't mastered.[55]

→ Chimpanzees easily best humans at recalling a set of numbers displayed for a fraction of a second.[56]

→ Crows can manufacture effective tools for fetching snacks from stuff they find lying around.[57] And we were told that tool making was one of the great *human* advancements of the Lower Paleolithic period. LOL.

→ Pigs are smarter than a three-year-old child. And last time I checked, we don't eat toddlers.[58]

→ Ants have complex social matriarchal communities in which male ants' sole jobs are to reproduce with and protect the queen.[59] If that ain't advancement beyond Western civilization's misogynistic norms, I don't know what is.

→ Rats are capable of complex interpersonal and extra-species bonds. They've been known to form friendships, pine when those bonds are lost or someone passes away, and, when tickled, make chirping sounds strikingly similar to human laughter.[60]

→ Cats. Look, anyone who's spent time around them knows they're manipulative as fuck, which takes intelligence. Not many studies about cat smarts have been conducted, however, because let's be real, cats are uncooperative and don't do anything they don't wanna do.[61]

→ Fish: not actually swimming vegetables. Five hundred–plus studies have shown that fish not only feel pain but have incredible memories that exceed those of "higher" vertebrates, including nonhuman primates.[62] Also, they're usually the best characters in Disney movies.

Hell, even slime mold, which is essentially an amoeba, has been found to have decision-making capabilities.[63] The point here is that nonhuman animals have dope abilities that are either crazy amazing compared to our own (supersonic hearing, panoramic vision, eight tits) or wildly similar to qualities and behaviors humans value (affection, community, empathy, a sense of humor). Before we starkly compartmentalize them as either friends or food, let's remember that animals, great and small, are unique creatures with important ecological contributions deserving of our respect. And if you still subscribe to the whole "we're at the top of the food chain, bro" racket, may I (1) put you in a cage with a hungry lion, and (2) invoke Gandhi's "the true measure of any society can be found in how it treats its most vulnerable members"? If you believe humans are the evolutionary heads of the animal kingdom, then I hope you also believe what's true of all good leaders—that it's incumbent upon us not to exploit but to protect.

MY REASONS?

As you've gathered from my charming high school graduation party story, I have not always eaten compassionately, and boy, do I understand that change—especially in the culture and pleasure center–influenced realm of food—can be scary and difficult. I didn't make this shift overnight (and I fucked up quite a bit along the way), and I certainly don't expect you to either. For me, it started with some dancing chickens. I'm not a huge woo-woo New-Age kind of person, but I believe in karma in some form. You know, the whole "we reap what we sow" business. The reality of what I was eating hit me when I saw a video of chickens listening to music. Like, no shit, these cluckers, feathers blowing in the wind, were bebopping to Chopin, blinking their eyes with contentment at every crescendo and scratching their little chicken claws on the ground with every beat like they were at a freaking honkytonk. That short video clip completely fucked with my reality. Like, why was I eating a creature that had a face, a mom, and, on top of all that, probably better musical taste than most of the people I'd dated? There came a point for me (and it may or may not for you, but fingers crossed for the former) when I had to align my generic "Squeeee! I love animals!" ethos with what it really means to love and respect all animals. Regardless of whether you're to that point, if you are serious about developing greener habits, there's no better place to knock it out of the park than in the kitchen.

The Ick Factor

I know some people for whom the transition to being vegan was ridiculously easy. Why? They had the ingrained yuck response to meat. And for good reason. Meat can be contaminated with feces, blood, and other bodily fluids; can be rife with potentially harmful antibiotics and medicines; and, according to the USDA, accounts for 70 percent of American food poisoning cases.[64] In fact, eight of the twelve items the US Food and Drug Administration (FDA) recommends persons with compromised immune systems (like children, pregnant women, and the elderly) avoid are animal products.[65]

The Solution Is So Freaking Simple

This is the part where I reveal that—SURPRISE!—eating fewer animal products is the freaking simplest solution to all the depressing info you just ugly cried through. Here's more feel-good news to sweeten the deal: it's estimated that a vegan diet produces 50 percent less carbon dioxide (that's more payoff than switching to an electric car!), uses one-eleventh the oil, one-thirteenth the water, and one-eighteenth the land, and saves one hundred–plus animals every year than eating meaty.[66] If you're more into taking it day by day, that's an estimated eleven hundred gallons of water, forty-five pounds of grain, thirty square feet of forested land, twenty pounds of CO_2, and one animal's life—for ONE DAY of eschewing animal products.[67] And you don't need to go whole hog. When compared to omnivorous eating, vegetarian diets have been shown to reduce

CO_2 emissions by 63 percent, and even tapered animal-product consumption can cut emissions by 29 percent.[68] Whatever reasons resonate most with you, explore them as you embrace one delicious veg-based meal at a time. And hey, there's no deadline here. No timer. No referee. No judge. No standard of purity or perfection. Do what feels right, exciting, and nourishing for you. I'm proud of you already, champ.

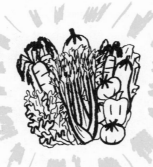

PUTTING IT INTO PRACTICE

No matter the cadence of your transition to eating more plant-based foods, there are plenty of simple habits you can adopt right freaking now related to food shopping and storage that will save you major bucks, reduce food and packaging waste, and make stocking your home for dietary success simple and stress-free. These tips will set you up for eco-success, whether you're slowly sashaying into a more vegan diet or have been instantly transformed into an overnight vegetarian. Regardless of your dietary preferences, you can employ some or all (wahoo!) of these steps to make grocery shopping a sustainable venture rather than the wasteful, expensive, frown-making drudgery it often is.

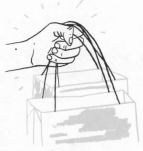

Food Shopping

BYOB: One of the easiest ways to reduce your footprint when you shop is to bring your own kit. This can be as simple or as complex as you like, depending upon the amount of waste you'd like to reduce, but be sure to start with the easiest thing you can do pretty much ever, which is to bring your own freaking bag. Plastic bags are the fourth most abundant item of trash, to the tune of one hundred billion bags used each year in America alone. Just the amount of oil required to manufacture these bags is enough to drive a car around the earth three times (approximately seventy-five thousand miles).[69] Old ladies are doing it. Your asshole neighbor who revs his motorbike at 2 a.m. does it. You should probably be doing it, man. Here's a primer for a little shopping kit you can put together that won't cost you much or weigh you down but will graduate you to grocery shopping the Give a Shit way:

→ Cloth shopping bags (I like canvas because they're washable and sturdy)

→ Cloth food bags in varying sizes (for vegetables and nuts)

→ Glass jars and bottles in various sizes (for bulk shopping)

→ Reusable dry erase marker, wax pencil, or washable crayon to mark bulk items

→ The Bulk Finder app from Zero Waste Home to find where items are sold in bulk near you

Know before you go: Avoid duplicative purchases by snapping a photo of your fridge and pantry before hitting the store. You'll free up brain space and be able to answer burning questions like "Do we already have pickles?" Answer: yes, but you can never have too many pickles.

Shop with a list: Although spontaneity is fun in the bedroom, it's a killer when it comes to sticking to a shopping budget and value system. And we've all been there—trapsein' into Target to get a last-minute lemon, only to leave with a duvet cover, picture frame, whisk, and Michael Buble's holiday CD. If you're a once-a-week mega shopper, do like Santa and make a list (I like the AnyList app), check it twice, and stay nice by sticking to it.

Buy only what you need: Stockpiling perishable food in your fridge is a recipe for mega-waste and probably a key criterion for candidacy on *Hoarders: Buried Alive*. If possible, do like the Europeans and do little shops every few days, building meals around what's fresh, in season, and in quantities you'll actually consume.

Grab organic when you can: Organic crops are grown without the synthetic fertilizers and pesticides used in conventional farming, thereby preserving the nutrients and microbial activity that keep soil healthy. Organic crops usually also yield more profit for farmers. Although it's not always possible to purchase organic, for your health, try to at least go organic when nabbing "dirty dozen" items like apples, peaches, and tomatoes.

Support fair trade: You may think of fair trade as a designation only for clothing, but 60 percent of the fair-trade market is food products. Why? Well, many items like coffee, tea, cocoa and chocolate, honey, bananas, and other produce come from countries where child and slave labor, nonlivable wages, and hazardous working conditions are the norm. Purchasing certified fair trade whenever possible supports more ethical labor standards, eco-friendly practices, and positive community development.

Avoid palm oil: Once you start reading labels, you'll be surprised how many items contain palm oil. In addition to being considered less nutritive than other oils, palm oil is a leading cause of deforestation and animal suffering. Orangutans, native to Borneo and Sumatra, are intelligent, gentle, totally rad, and classified as endangered. They also suffer greatly to meet our rapidly increasing palm oil demands. Their rainforest habitats are cleared at the rate of three hundred football fields per hour to make way for monoculture palm oil plantations, and it's estimated that five hundred thousand orangutans have been slaughtered as agricultural pests in the past twenty years.[70] At this rate endangered orangutans will likely be extinct within ten to twenty years.[71] You can avoid palm oil by scouring food and personal care labels (it's especially present in beauty and cleaning products, nut butters, processed snack bars, candy, crackers, chocolate, margarine, and ice cream), dodging products that don't specify the contents of oil blends, and eschewing processed items in favor of homemade versions. I love you, orangutans.

Eat "ugly" food: From farm to fork, 52 percent of all produce in the United States goes uneaten.[72] Because we've been influenced by marketing to believe that unnaturally flawless, often genetically modified fruits and veggies are cleaner and healthier, less cosmetically appealing produce often hits the trash before it ever reaches the store. Less-than-perfect items taste the same (and sometimes better, as they tend to be organic heirloom varieties that are bursting with flavor) and can save you money. Opt for delicious ugly ducklings when you're at the farmers' market or grocery store, and explore local subscription services and community-supported agriculture (CSA) dedicated to giving imperfect produce their day in the sun.

WATCH YOUR MOUTH

Selecting the safest produce can sometimes feel like a battle. Never fear, friend, the Environmental Working Group's annual Shopper's Guide to Pesticides in Produce is here.[v] See, these nice folks look at the US Department of Agriculture's Pesticide Data Program report and determine the "Dirty Dozen" (produce more likely to be contaminated with crazy shit like pesticide residue) and "Clean 15" (produce less likely to absorb pesticides).[vi] Feast your eyes on these, and whenever possible opt for organic or local, nonpesticide versions of the Double D's (mind out of the gutter, guys).

The Dirty Dozen

1. Strawberries
2. Spinach
3. Nectarines
4. Apples
5. Peaches
6. Celery
7. Grapes
8. Pears
9. Cherries
10. Tomatoes
11. Sweet bell peppers
12. Potatoes

The Clean 15

1. Sweet corn
2. Avocados
3. Pineapples
4. Cabbage
5. Onions
6. Frozen sweet peas
7. Papayas
8. Asparagus
9. Mangoes
10. Eggplant
11. Honeydew
12. Kiwifruit
13. Cantaloupe
14. Cauliflower
15. Grapefruit

Reduce packaging: You know what's cool? Food that comes from the earth often has its own biodegradable wrappers. Fruits and vegetables don't need to be doubly cloaked in plastic cling film, and dried beans and nuts don't taste better when they're sold in paper boxes with cellophane panes. When shopping, look for the least amount of packaging possible, and if packaging is unavoidable, go for the largest quantity available in recyclable or reusable containers. Moreover, when selecting produce, pick the ones without those pesky stickers. Although some companies are tinkering with biodegradable paper versions and tattoos, traditional stickers are noncompostable or recyclable plastic, though oddly the FDA says they're safe to eat (WUT).[73]

Buy in bulk: No, not the big-box kind of bulk shopping that has you schlepping fifty mini-bags of pretzels. I'm talking those bins at health food and grocery stores where you can buy the same premium nonperishables you typically purchase packaged, but when buying in bulk you get it for 15 to 30 percent less dough.[74] If you buy beans, legumes, seeds, nuts, grains, nut butters, coffee, tea, granola, spices, dry baking stuff, dried fruit, or candy, you can spare the planet unnecessary packaging whilst saving an estimated $100-plus a month by switching to bulk. Some places even offer cleaning and grooming products; cooking liquids like maple syrup, oils, vinegars, and soy sauce; and pet supplies in bulk. And if you're worried that bulk items are less sanitary than their packaged counterparts, think again. The FDA allows for certain particle percentages in all packaged and processed goods. What kinds of particles? As an example, six subsamples of macaroni and noodle products are allowed to contain 225 insect fragments (arms, legs, antennae) or four and a half rodent hairs or excreta (that's feces, guys) per 225 grams.[75] So ready your refillables and prepare to save big on everything from organics to spices.

Stay local: Farmers' markets are the best places to buy high-quality, local, in-season, minimally packaged food. Make it a weekly ritual, get to know your vendors (they always have the best recipes), and experiment with new-to-you foods. In addition to the usual fresh fare, my local market sells artisan breads, vinegars, cold-brew coffee, kombucha, loose-leaf tea blends, tofu and miso, package-free snacks like vegan pierogis and tamales, homemade soaps and lotions, pet treats, pasta, gorgeous plants and flowers, and one-of-a-kind ceramics. It's basically heaven. Find your local markets via the USDA's Farmers Market Directory, and also consider CSA options. Many local farms will deliver produce, bread, and other goodies right to your door with an affordable subscription. Your food will be fresher and travel fewer miles, while you not only support small businesses and responsible agricultural practices but also eat exciting seasonal vittles.

Walk and haul: This may sound arduous to those who are habituated to loading up the SUV and heading to Costco, but if you're buying food to last for a few days at a time, this method is extremely helpful in ensuring you get only what you need. I started doing this when I lived in Boston after graduate school. I was broke as a joke, had no ride (and this was before the advent of ride sharing), and lived in a fourth-floor walk-up. I would trot to my local grocery store and, because I had to haul everything back home on foot, eschew buying items that had crazy packaging and heavy liquids. For instance, a bouillon cube has a smaller footprint than a big package of broth, and loose tea you brew at home (just add water!)

is way greener than bottled versions. You can certainly abide by those tenets if you drive to the store, but sometimes it's nice to have a very physical reminder to keep your habits in check.

Shop the perimeter: You can still be eco-friendly if your only shopping option is a traditional grocery store with no bulk aisle. Avoiding egregious packaging (and buying generally healthier, less processed food) is easier when you stick to the perimeter of the store. And because many items at traditional grocery stores have loads of packaging, do your best to lighten the ecological load by buying items in recyclable packaging. For instance, a large plastic clamshell of spinach might seem way worse for the environment than the light, smaller plastic bag of spinach, but that bag can't be recycled, so clamshell is the way to go. Just do your best and be thoughtful. You've already got a gold star in my book, kid.

Store properly: You know what isn't good for food freshness? Sitting in a sweltering car or hanging out in the bag while you dick around on your Xbox. When you get home from shopping, prioritize properly storing your food so it stays fresher longer.

Prep ASAP: Do you ever get home from a grueling day at work, look at the giant watermelon on your counter or head of cauliflower in your crisper and say, "Fuck it. Nothing to eat," before dialing your local Chinese delivery place? Yes, me too. But if that watermelon is cut into juicy cubes and that cauliflower is already rubbed with aromatic curry and roasted to savory perfection, you're going to chowtown instead of copping to end-of-day laziness. Bottom line: Meal prep is a rad way to prevent food waste. Cut the carrots, make the soup, brew the tea, and pack it up (along with your tired excuses) for easy access during the busy week. Need inspiration? Here come some recipes (yay!), but first . . . another story (you know you love 'em).

Mo' Recipes, Mo' Problems

The first year of being vegan, I subsisted almost entirely on smoothies, Vegenaise, and Chick'n Tenders. Oh, and delicious, delicious blueberry vodka sodas. Like, I shit you not, that was the lion's share of my grocery list. See, the issue wasn't that I didn't know how to cook but rather that I was stymied by the sheer volume of recipes out there. I would thumb through cookbooks, dog-ear the shit out of them, and, then, do nothing. It wasn't that these books weren't chock full of everything I could ever want to eat and the appropriate guidance on how to make 'em, it was that I (1) wanted to make everything and (2) could never seem to find the time. #FirstWorldProblems

So I'm not going to overwhelm you with hundreds of recipes. There are loads of gorgeous, food porn–laden cookbooks written by talented souls that will teach you how to mill your own flour, make vegan cheese from scratch, and sprout beans and things. Pick those up for sure, but I have a hunch you selected this book because you want the easiest and most pain-free route to get from point A (where you are now) to point B (eco-nirvana) in your metaphorical hybrid car.

Instead, I'm gonna do you a solid and give you just the recipes you need to effortlessly slay the actual life situations that crop up. Whether you need a dish to wow the smug, perfectly coiffed PTA moms, an eye- and mouth-gasm that'll have people begging for seconds at a potluck, something quick and tasty to bring for not-sad desk lunches, or an impressive spread to inspire *l'amour*, I've got you covered with these uncomplicated, mind-blowingly delish, affordable, totally indispensable recipes that will help you make the kitch your bitch. Moreover, every recipe ingredient features symbols to indicate eco-friendly disposal, if any, so you can repurpose, recycle, and compost with confidence.

And if you're concerned that eating in this way is going to be boring, well, you picked up the wrong book, homie. My appreciation for good food runs deep, and my travels have cultivated a taste for well-balanced cuisines with just a touch of the exotic to keep things interesting. Prepare for the unexpected visitors and party invites to roll in, you sexy thang.

PLANT-BASED RECIPES
TO GET YOUR GRUB ON

DON'T BE TRASHY

Sometimes you gotta know when to hold 'em and when to fold 'em. Or, in the case of this book, know when to recycle 'em and when to compost 'em. For every ingredient herein, I give you a little symbol indicating how to dispose of the leftover stuff. Whether it's repurposing or recycling an aluminum can, saving onion tops so you can make the dopest vegetable broth of your life, or composting scraps, I'll never leave you with a pile of trash. And that's a promise.

[RP] *Repurpose (containers and packaging)*

[RC] *Recycle (containers and packaging)*

[S] *Save (food to use in other recipes)*

[C] *Compost (food and other bio-degradable materials)*

Peep each recipe's Clean-Up Notes for the skinny on how to ethically off-load ingredients.

Serious Staples

Okay, I know I just waxed poetic about how I'm not going to show you how to make a bunch of complicated stuff, but I do need to spill on a few recipes that will become indispensable in your arsenal of plant-based cooking. Making these yourself will not only save you the big bucks and up your eco-cred but will also taste way better than store-bought stuff.

WHITE WITCH ALMOND MILK

The creamy, alabaster
elixir of the gods

Whether it's crowning your morning coffee, cascading over your granola, or making a splash in a cold glass, almond milk is the white witch of plant-based cooking. Once you have this recipe down, you can make variations to your heart's content and delight at eschewing the additives and wasteful packaging of store-bought versions. Because this recipe is free from said preservatives and thickeners commonly used in store-bought versions, I recommend consuming within about three days. Moreover, homemade almond milk has an unparalleled richness and flavor you'll come to love. Prefer cashews, walnuts, pecans, pistachios, pumpkin seeds? Get crazy with 'em. Want to make a coconut, banana, or cocoa-laden variety? Get stupid with it. Just be sure to store in a glass container and shake before using to break up the natural almond-y goodness that can separate and settle at the bottom.

——————————— *Makes 4 cups* ———————————

Prep time: 5 minutes
Total time: 1 to 10 hours
(depending on how long you want to soak your nuts)

1½ cups raw almonds

3 cups water for soaking, plus 4 cups water for milk

2 (or more, to taste) Medjool dates, pitted

½ teaspoon vanilla extract

Pinch sea salt, to taste

Cheesecloth, for straining
(preferably 100% unbleached cotton) or a fine mesh strainer

Soak the almonds: Place the almonds in a bowl, and pour over enough cold water to cover; soak overnight, about 8 to 10 hours, or, if you're pinched for time, soak for an hour in hot water. Drain the liquid from the almonds and rinse well.

Prepare the milk: Place the drained and rinsed almonds, 4 cups water, dates, vanilla, and salt in a high-speed blender, and blend on the highest speed for 1 minute or slightly longer to get the desired creaminess.

Strain: Hold a cheesecloth bag or strainer over a large bowl, and slowly pour the almond milk mixture into the bag or strainer. Give the bag a good squeeze to release any additional milk from the pulp. Repeat the process as necessary to achieve the desired thickness and remove any lingering almond bits.

Decant the milk: Into a glass bottle, and store in the fridge for up to 3 days. Use on everything.

CLEAN-UP NOTES:

[S] Almond meal (the pulp that's left in your cheesecloth after you've strained the milk). Allow to dry and freeze in a glass container for use in smoothies, baking recipes, and oatmeal for an extra punch of healthy fiber, or use in making homemade skin scrubs.

[C] Cheesecloth

[RP] White Witch Almond Milk: this may sound wacky, but if you can't finish this ambrosia before its shelf life is up, make like Cleopatra and consider putting it in your bath as a nutritive soak.

OTHER BADASS VARIETIES

If you want some cool variations, here are some I rock on the regular, just be sure to consume at the peak of freshness, about 1 to 2 days after making:

Lavender-Vanilla Almond Milk: Add ½ teaspoon lavender buds and half a vanilla bean (with the seeds scooped out and stirred into the milk, along with the empty bean) to the finished almond milk bottle. Let them infuse in the milk for a few hours (or overnight for more potency) until it's reached your desired level of flavor, and then strain out and compost the lavender buds and vanilla pod.

Salted Chocolate Almond Milk: Add 3 tablespoons quality cocoa powder (or cacao powder if you prefer), 1 tablespoon maple syrup, and 1 teaspoon extra sea salt (or more, to taste) to the blender when you add the other ingredients.

Chai Spice Almond Milk: Add 1 chai tea bag to your almond milk and allow to steep in the fridge for 4 hours to overnight, depending on desired potency. This is freaking amazing in homemade chai and in iced lattes, BTW.

HUMMUS-SAPIEN

*When your entire person is
comprised of hummus*

It doesn't matter who you are, how you eat, or where you're from—it's been scientifically proven that everyone on the planet loves hummus. Think about it: Have you ever met a person who hates hummus? Didn't think so. Making your own is not only less expensive (seriously, store-bought hummus? $7 for 6 ounces? WTF?) and lighter on packaging, but it tastes so much freaking better. An Israeli friend in grad school who was so tired of seeing us all make garbage hummus ("You guys make it too lemony, too garlicky!") taught me this recipe. The flavor is decidedly more mild than the overly spiced and citric hummus we're accustomed to and I am here for it. If using dry chickpeas, the process takes a little more time, but it's very worth it for the richest, silkiest hummus of your life. And if you don't have that kind of time, this recipe still makes canned chickpeas sing. No, this is not a romance novel, but it could be.

Makes 8 servings
(or 1, if you're me and hungover)

Prep time: 30 minutes
**Total time: 30 minutes if using canned chickpeas,
1 day if using dry chickpeas**

INGREDIENTS

1 cup dried chickpeas or 1 (15-ounce) can

2 teaspoons baking soda, if using dry chickpeas

6-7 large garlic cloves, unpeeled

1 medium lemon, juiced (about ¼ cup)

½ cup tahini, room temperature
and stirred

¼ cup olive oil

½ teaspoon ground cumin

1 teaspoon soy sauce

Salt and pepper, to taste

Optional: Smoked paprika, freshly chopped parsley,
extra olive oil for serving

IF USING DRY CHICKPEAS:

Soak the chickpeas: Place chickpeas in a bowl and cover with cold water (by about 4 inches). Add half the baking soda (1 teaspoon) and allow to soak at room temperature (just cover the bowl with a clean dish cloth) overnight.

Once soaked, drain the excess liquid and rinse chickpeas with cold water.

Cook chickpeas and garlic: In a pot, add the soaked chickpeas, unpeeled garlic cloves, remaining baking soda, and 3 cups of water and bring to a boil over high heat. Reduce to medium-high heat and let simmer until chickpeas are soft, about 1 to 1½ hours.

Make the liquid: While chickpeas are cooking, combine the lemon juice, tahini, olive oil, cumin, and soy sauce together in a bowl until smooth.

Remove the skins: Once chickpeas are very tender (according to my friend, slightly overcooked chickpeas are key for creamy hummus), drain, reserving ½ cup of the cooking water. Now you have a choice: you can remove the chickpea skins (by lightly pinching chickpeas to free the meat from the skin) or leave them on. Remove the garlic skins and place the chickpeas (peeled or unpeeled), peeled garlic, and tahini mixture in the food processor.

Blend the humus: Pulse, scraping down the sides, to ensure everything is combined, adding the reserved cooking liquid as you go until desired consistency is reached.

Add salt and pepper to taste.

IF USING CANNED CHICKPEAS:

Cook chickpeas and garlic: Drain and save the liquid from the can (lovingly called aquafaba, which can be saved in a glass jar in the fridge to make amazing whipped cream and other wonders). Rinse the chickpeas well.

In a small saucepan, add the unpeeled garlic cloves and 2 cups water and bring to a boil over high heat. Reduce to medium-high heat and let simmer until garlic cloves are tender, about 30 minutes.

Make the liquid: While garlic cloves are cooking, combine the lemon juice, tahini, olive oil, cumin, and soy sauce together in a bowl until smooth.

Remove the skins: Once garlic cloves are tender, drain, reserving ½ cup of the cooking water. Remove the skins.

Blend the hummus: Place the chickpeas, peeled garlic, and tahini mixture in the food processor. Pulse, scraping down the sides, to ensure everything is combined, adding the reserved cooking liquid bit by bit as you go until desired consistency is reached. Pulse and regularly check consistency—remember, liquid can always be added but cannot be taken away!

Salt and pepper to taste.

As hummus is a matter of taste, feel free to add more lemon juice, a fresh garlic clove, or other spices after you've blended the base mixture. I've come to love the simple richness of this recipe as it is. Spread into a bowl and garnish with a sprinkle (½ teaspoon) smoked paprika, a drizzle of olive oil, and fresh parsley.

CLEAN-UP NOTES

[S] Aquafaba: for making cool shit like meringues and whipped cream (see the Jamocha Silk Pie on page 168) and for use in anything that needs thickening or whipping.

[S] Garlic peels: for use in Scrap-Happy Broth (page 136)

[S] Lemon peel: add to Infused Cleaning Vinegar.

[C] Chickpea skins (if using dried)

[RP] Chickpea can: clean and repurpose as a cute pen cup, makeup brush holder, or telephone game.

OTHER BADASS VARIETIES

If you want some cool variations, here are ones I rock on the regular:

Jalapeño Lime Hummus: Dice a jalapeño (remove the seeds and connective tissue if you don't want too much heat) and stir (don't blend!) half the jalapeño into the hummus. Add a few tablespoons of fresh lime juice to taste.

Garnish with diced purple onion, the remaining diced jalapeño, and fresh cilantro. Pair with tortilla chips, and pig out.

Pickle Hummus: People may point and laugh at you for saying you're eating pickle hummus, but those people don't matter because this hummus is KING. Finely dice three full dill pickles and fold into hummus with 1 to 2 tablespoons of pickle liquid to taste. Chop fresh dill and fold in to taste. Top with more fresh dill and lots of coarsely ground black pepper. This pairs extremely well with kettle-cooked potato chips and a cold beer.

Bombay Hummus: This is a lovely marriage of two of my favorite cuisines. Add 1 teaspoon garam masala, ½ teaspoon madras curry powder, and freshly chopped cilantro to taste. Pair with naan or chapati for a spiritual experience.

Persian Hummus: Fold 1 tablespoon za'tar and 1 tablespoon lime juice to taste. Top with roasted pistachios and pomegranate seeds for an exotic twist. This pairs beautifully with crisped pita bread.

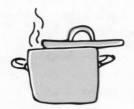

SCRAP-HAPPY BROTH

Once you go scrap, you never go back

Throughout my journey to lower-waste living, few things have tormented me more than the regret I feel for not having invented scrap broth. So dang simple and genius, it's truly a utilitarian idea laid by the gods. This broth is a versatile addition to soups, sauces, and cooking liquid for grains and legumes and for sautéing in lieu of oil. Simply keep a bag (I used an old ziplock I keep washing and reusing) or container in your freezer, and whenever you're prepping veggies, get in the habit of tossing the tops, tips, skins, and leftovers in the bag. Just don't add cucumbers, spinach and kale, cruciferous veggies like broccoli and Brussels sprouts, radishes, and gloppier veggies like tomatoes and eggplant in this broth because they can impart a weird bitterness that's no bueno. Also, never add rotten or moldy veggies to the broth—if you wouldn't eat it, don't put it in your broth! Best to just compost anything that's well past its prime. If you're pressed for time, you can skip the roasting step and add your scraps and ingredients straight to a soup pot for longer simmering. I like to enjoy this broth with a hearty dollop of miso, freshly diced jalapeño, and green onion. It's your broth, so get crazy with it!

Makes about 8 to 9 cups

Prep time: 10 minutes
Total time: 2 to 3 hours (most of which doesn't involve you at all—relax)

INGREDIENTS

4 cups vegetable scraps

2 tablespoons white miso

2 tablespoons olive oil

3 garlic cloves, unpeeled

4–5 dried shiitake mushrooms

2 small sundried tomatoes

8–10 cups water, depending on the size of your pot
and desired broth richness

Salt and pepper, to taste

Optional:
2–3 tablespoons Bragg's Aminos
or soy sauce, to taste

Preheat oven to 300°F. If they're frozen, defrost your scraps a bit so you can break them up. Prepare a baking sheet with a Silpat liner or parchment paper.

Coat the scraps: In the scraps bag, add the miso, oil, and garlic; seal, then shake until the scraps are evenly coated. Spread the mixture evenly on the baking sheet, and roast until the vegetables are aromatic and shriveled, about 30 minutes to an hour, depending on the size of the scraps (smaller scraps can burn quickly, so watch them carefully!).

Prepare the broth: Transfer the roasted scraps to a soup pot, add the dried mushrooms and sundried tomatoes, and cover with water to nearly the top of the pot. Bring to a boil, then reduce heat, cover, and simmer for an hour.

After the hour, taste the broth. If you want more umami flavor, add the Bragg's Aminos or soy sauce to taste. Finish with salt and pepper as desired.

Strain the liquid: Pour the broth through a mesh strainer, squeezing every bit of juice from the scraps, and decant into glass jars, allowing it to cool to room temperature before putting on the lids.

This broth can be stored in the fridge for up to 1½ weeks or in the freezer for up to 6 months. If freezing, do not overfill glass jars as liquid expands as it transforms into a solid state.

CLEAN-UP NOTES

[C] Strained vegetable scraps, parchment paper (if unwaxed)

The Everyday Slay

Quick breakfasts, make-ahead lunches, and meals you'll be excited to whip together, even after a long day—these nourishing and comforting recipes are sure to become part of your daily arsenal.

GET-YOUR-SHIT-TOGETHER SMOOTHIE

A good-for-you habit that tastes like dessert

The advice to "eat your greens" certainly is sage, but busy schedules and general brattiness on our part can make adulting hard. That's why I try to front-load as many greens as possible early in the day (mostly so I can feel better about cocktails and fries later). It's a wise strategy because you hydrate and nourish (also known as "getting one's shit together") in one easy sip. Full disclosure: I feel a little silly including a smoothie recipe because, well, it's a smoothie. There's not much culinary science behind it. But this one is delish (it seriously tastes like vanilla ice cream) and won't break the bank, so it's a staple I had to include. Use the optional add-ins to customize to your personal taste and needs, and create a gorgeous green guzzler you'll feel totally baller walking into work with.

Makes 2 servings
(I bring any remaining for lunch or a snack)

Total time: 5 minutes

INGREDIENTS

1 medium banana, peeled and frozen
(I peel and freeze a ton in advance so I always have some on hand)

1 cup fresh or frozen pineapple chunks

Big handful baby spinach, about 1½ cups

2 cups White Witch Almond Milk (page 130,
the Chai Spice version really makes this next level, BTW)
or nut milk of choice

2 pitted Medjool dates

½ teaspoon cinnamon

¼ teaspoon ground ginger

1 teaspoon vanilla extract

Optional:
1 teaspoon vanilla plant-based protein powder,
spirulina, or chlorella powder for extra green goodness,
or 1 tablespoon almond meal left over from making
White Witch Almond Milk for an extra punch of fiber

Put all of that shit in a high-speed blender, and whir until smooth. Add more almond milk until desired thickness is achieved. And get crazy with this—sub orange juice, coconut water, or pineapple juice for the almond milk to get different flavors. Pour it into two Mason jars (if you're feelin' twee), and enjoy with a friend or keep the second for a postworkout pick-me-up or sippable snack.

CLEAN-UP NOTES

[C] Banana peels

MORNING PERSON MORSELS

The grab-and-go brekkie that's like
a spicy-sweet alarm clock for your mouth

Every new year I write a resolution to "become a morning person." You know, those early risers who log an eight-mile jog with their pooch, a meditation and gratitude journaling session, a hearty breakfast, intensive goal setting, and pageant-perfect grooming all before 7:30 a.m.? I deeply want to be like those people. I also really, really like to stay up late, dance to New Wave in my jammies, sleep hard, and hit the snooze button. These densely delish and nutrish morsels (cookies, really), which were a happy accident when dicking around with the pulp from the White Witch Almond Milk, mean that I've at least got the "hearty breakfast" part down. And now you will too. They're also a perfectly tasty take-along for a party. You're welcome.

Makes 24 small-ish cookies

Prep time: 20 minutes
Total time: 30 minutes

INGREDIENTS

2 cups raw almonds

1 cup all-purpose gluten-free flour

½ teaspoon salt, to taste

2 tablespoons cinnamon

1 to 2 chai tea bags, opened (about 1–2 tablespoons loose tea),
depending on your preference

⅓ cup coconut oil, melted

1 teaspoon vanilla extract

½ teaspoon fresh orange zest, minced

½ cup maple syrup

Preheat your oven to 350°F and prepare two cookie sheets with parchment or Silpat liners.

Mill the almonds: In a high-speed blender with a dry blade, add the dry, raw almonds and mill in to a dry almond meal. You can choose the consistency (I like a slightly crunchy consistency because it adds a nice chewy texture to these cookies). In a large bowl, add milled almond meal with the flour, salt, cinnamon, and chai tea bag contents to taste (if you don't *love* chai, go for just one bag, and add more after the dough has been made).

Prepare the liquid: In a smaller bowl blend melted coconut oil, vanilla extract, and orange zest. Add maple syrup to liquid mixture. (Psst: This mixture will smell like heaven.)

Mix the batter: Once stirred, gently fold liquid into dry mixture with a spatula.

The dough should be slightly sticky, but firm enough to form into balls. This is when I taste the dough to see if it has the right amount of salt for my liking.

Roll the dough: Begin pinching dough and rolling into Ping-Pong ball–sized balls (this recipe yields about 24) and arrange on baking sheets. This is a sticky job, but focus on using the palm of your hands instead of the fingers. Push down slightly on the cookies to flatten a bit, but leave some volume, which will keep them thick and chewy. Make sure to evenly space out cookies so they all bake independently of one another.

Bake the morsels: Place cookie sheets in oven and set a timer for 8 minutes (be sure to check the bottoms of your cookies after 8 minutes, as these bad boys can burn if not watched). In some ovens, the cookies will be done at 8 minutes, or they might need up to 2 minutes more. When the bottoms of the cookies start to look more brown than the tops, your cookies are done.

Cool and serve: Remove from oven and place on cooling rack. Wait until these puppies cool to taste them. The wait will be worth it.

CLEAN-UP NOTES

[C] Tea bags (if compostable and if not using non-loose tea), parchment paper (if unwaxed)

[S] Orange: add to Infused Cleaning Vinegar, or use in Tropical Quinoa Tabbouleh (page 142)

TROPICAL QUINOA
TABBOULEH

*The perfect take-along lunch for when you want
everyone to think you're a cool model*

You know that girl at work who takes delicate bites of a salad while you're chowing down on loaded potato skins? We secretly envy that girl, but it's only because we secretly kind of want to be her (or, at least, to have her BYO savvy). This salad makes it easy to be a cool-girl bringer of salads. It's loaded with fiber-rich greens, protein-packed quinoa, juicy fruit, and a dressing that will make you want to make out with strangers (if you don't already wrestle with that urge). I like to make a double batch and then dish servings into individual glass containers so I have kick-ass lunches for the week.

Makes 2 servings

Total time: 30 minutes

INGREDIENTS

¾ cup quinoa

1 cup canned pineapple chunks, diced,
with juice reserved, divided

1½ cups water

1 medium lime, halved and ¼ teaspoon zested

Salt and pepper, to taste

⅓ cup finely diced red onion

4 cups kale, stems and ribs removed, chopped

¼ cup apple cider vinegar

1 tablespoon maple syrup

½ cup raw cashews

1 navel orange, deseeded and diced,
and 1 teaspoon zested

1 tablespoon finely chopped fresh mint leaves

Cook the quinoa: In a saucepan, combine the quinoa, ¼ cup of the pineapple juice, water, juice of half the lime, and a dash of salt. Bring to a boil, then reduce heat to a low simmer, and cook for 15 to 20 minutes, or until all the liquid is absorbed. Once it's tender, fluff it with a fork, remove from heat, salt and pepper to taste, and allow it to chill in the refrigerator.

Massage the kale: In a large bowl, add the red onion, kale, and the remaining lime juice. Using your hands, massage the lime juice into the kale to tenderize and remove bitterness, about 1 minute.

Prepare the dressing: In a small jar or bowl, combine the vinegar, remaining pineapple juice, maple syrup, and the lime zest.

Toast the cashews: In a dry sauté pan, place the cashews, and toast them over low-medium heat for 5 minutes, stirring to ensure they don't burn. The cashews toast quickly and are done when they emit a roasted aroma and are lightly browned. Remove them from the pan, and set aside.

Assemble the tabbouleh: Add the quinoa to the bowl with the kale and onion. Fold in the orange, mint, pineapple chunks, and lime and orange zest to taste. Add the dressing and salt and pepper to taste. Ladle into a dish, and garnish with cashews, if desired.

If you're packing this dish to go, keep the dressing and cashews separate and add when you're ready to chow down.

CLEAN-UP NOTES

[S] Mint and parsley stems: use for infusing iced tea with fresh flavor

[S] Onion skins and tops: for Scrap-Happy Broth

[S] Orange, lime peels: for Infused Cleaning Vinegar

[RP] Pineapple can: clean and repurpose

[C] Kale stems

PICNIC-PERFECT
PANZANELLA

Prayers are answered:
A salad made almost entirely from bread

Now, this is a salad I can really get behind! Bursting with fresh ingredients you can easily buy sans packaging (this is especially wonderful in the summer when fresh tomatoes abound), this recipe boasts near-effortless preparation and flavors that get better the longer they mingle. So, if you're that rare species who happens to have bread in your house that you have not eaten immediately (seriously, who the fuck are you and can you teach me your ways?), this "salad" (air quotes) is pretty much the ideal place for said bread to go. Even if it's wicked stale (if that's the case, wrap it in a clean, damp dishcloth and zap it in the microwave for 30 seconds, or in a 350°F oven for 10 minutes or until it softens). Plus, you can jazz this up as you'd like. Contrary to my grandmother's not-so-popular belief, there are no Panzanella Police who are going to whack you with their baguette bully club if you use sourdough, add more tomatoes than bread, or toss in whatever fresh things (basil is a nice addition if you have it on hand) you think might taste dope in here. Make your salad without fear, friends.

———————— *Makes 4 servings* ————————

Prep time: 20 minutes
Total time: 1 hour (most of which is time
where this salad is chilling in the fridge)

INGREDIENTS

FOR THE SALAD:

1 tablespoon olive oil

1 clove garlic, minced

1 demi (meaning half the size of a regular baguette, kids)
French baguette, or any leftover bread of choice, about 4–5 cups
cut into ½–1" cubes (depending on your preference)

¼ teaspoon garlic powder

2 medium heirloom tomatoes, or 20 small grape tomatoes (really, you can't add too many tomatoes here), diced to be about the same size as the bread cubes

1 shallot, thinly sliced

FOR THE DRESSING:

¼ cup olive oil

2 tablespoons red wine vinegar

1 teaspoon Dijon mustard

Salt and pepper, to taste

Toast the bread: In a high-sided skillet, add the olive oil and garlic over high heat. Once fragrant, or after about 1 minute, add the cubed bread and the garlic powder and stir to coat the cubes. Lower heat and sauté, stirring occasionally to prevent burning, for 5 to 8 minutes, or until the bread is lightly toasted (you can add more olive oil if you need as you go, and don't stir too frequently so the bread develops a crunchy, delicious texture). Remove from heat once your bread is nice and toasty.

Make the dressing: In a jar, add the olive oil, red wine vinegar, and Dijon mustard. Tighten the lid and shake well. Add salt and pepper to taste. If you prefer, you can also whisk the dressing together in a bowl.

Mix the panzanella: In a large bowl, combine the sautéed bread, sliced tomatoes, and sliced shallot.

Add dressing to the bread mixture and toss to coat ingredients evenly. Add more salt and pepper to taste, if desired.

Chill and serve: Cover with a clean dishcloth and allow to marinate for at least an hour before serving. Garnish however you see fit (I like adding fresh basil in the summer for extra flavor and color!).

CLEAN-UP NOTES

[S] Shallot and garlic skins: for Scrap-Happy Broth

CRAZY CREAMY MAC & CHEESE

The one recipe you need to
bid dairy adieu forever

Listen, I've been vegan for a long time, and when I first went the way of the vegetable, I had a pretty tough time ditching dairy, mostly because cheese, yo. So, this was one of the first recipes I worked tirelessly to perfect because it was exactly the kind of mac and cheese I wanted to make. So many vegan mac recipes try to trick you with sweet potatoes and white beans and other things, and I was simply not having any of it. I wanted real, honest-to-goodness creaminess, richness, sharp cheesiness. And I have it on good authority by many non-vegan friends that this really hits the mark. Now, I do use a few packaged ingredients here because, well, I feel they make a big difference. And if that difference helps to keep you from hitting the cow teat every now and then, I call that a win for planet and palate. Also, this cheese sauce is oh-so-dope on other things (burgers, nachos, poured straight into your mouth), so make it and keep it on hand for cheese-craving emergencies.

Makes 6 servings
(but let's be real; you're gonna eat this
all in one sitting)

Total time: 30 minutes

INGREDIENTS

16 ounces macaroni (or any other) pasta

½ cup cashews, soaked and drained (for up to an hour in hot water, or overnight in cold water)

½ cup nutritional yeast

1 Daiya Jalapeño Havarti Style Farmhouse Block, diced

1 vegan bouillon cube

1 cup Scrap-Happy Broth or other vegetable broth

1 clove garlic, peeled and minced

1 teaspoon olive oil

1 tablespoon soy sauce

4 drops liquid smoke (or ½ teaspoon smoked salt if you can't find liquid smoke)

½ teaspoon smoked paprika

½ teaspoon turmeric

½ teaspoon onion powder

½ teaspoon dried basil

1 teaspoon lemon juice

Pinch of nutmeg, to taste

Salt and pepper, to taste

Green onion, finely diced

Cook pasta: In a large pot of boiling water, add a pinch of salt and your macaroni, and cook until al dente. Strain, reserving 1 cup of the pasta water, and set aside.

Prepare the sauce: While the pasta is cooking, combine the cashews, nutritional yeast, Daiya block, bouillon cube, and broth in a blender and blend until smooth. Add some of the reserved pasta water if needed while blending.

Finish the sauce: In the same pot you used to cook the pasta, sauté the olive oil and garlic clove over medium-high heat for 1 minute. Add the cheesy mixture, and reduce heat to medium-low, allowing to warm, stirring gently, for about 4 minutes. Once warmed, add the soy sauce, liquid smoke or smoked salt, paprika, turmeric, onion powder, and dried basil, tasting as you go to achieve desired richness of flavor. Add the lemon juice and a pinch of nutmeg to taste, and season with salt and pepper to taste. If needed, add some reserved pasta water to achieve desired consistency (the sauce should be creamy).

Assemble the mac: Add the cooked pasta to the pot, coating entirely. Allow to warm together for 1 minute and then plate, garnish with diced green onion, and enjoy.

CLEAN-UP NOTES

[S] Garlic skins, green onion scraps: for Scrap-Happy Broth

[S] Lemon: for Infused Cleaning Vinegar

WALNUT CHORIZO TOSTADAS

Basically my food boyfriend. Enough said.

When I make this for the week, I am ridiculously delighted to see the ingredients waiting for me, all deconstructed and ready to assemble into a masterpiece, when I arrive home after a long day. These crispy, savory, creamy mouthfuls of amazing will satiate any craving you have. They're loaded with rich smashed black beans, crunchy fresh veggies, spiced crema, and a homemade walnut chorizo that you'll want to marry. These also make dope party appetizers. Just skip the tortillas and go straight for shoveling these into corn chips, and your finger food wishes are granted. Enjoy with a cold beer, and dream of sandy beaches and naked people. Or make like me and chomp on these whilst in your pajamas, scrolling social media on your couch as your dog stares at you.

Makes 2 to 3 servings

Total time: 40 minutes

INGREDIENTS

1 cup walnuts, finely chopped

1 clove garlic, minced

1 tablespoon apple cider vinegar

¼ teaspoon cumin, divided

¼ teaspoon chili powder, divided

¼ teaspoon smoked paprika, divided

Salt and pepper, to taste

6 corn tortillas

1 tablespoon olive oil

1 (16-ounce) can black beans, drained and rinsed

½ cup salsa, divided

⅓ cup Vegenaise

1 lime, juiced

¼ cup pickled jalapeños, drained, juice reserved

1½ cups shredded lettuce

1 radish, thinly sliced into coin-shaped rounds

⅛ cup finely diced red onion

Preheat the oven to 400°F, and line a baking sheet with a Silpat liner or parchment paper.

Make the walnut chorizo: In a medium bowl, combine the walnuts, garlic, vinegar, cumin, chili powder, paprika, and salt and pepper to taste. Stir and mash together until the spices are evenly combined. Allow it to sit at room temperature for 10 minutes. Give thanks to the food gods that you have discovered this amazingness.

Toast the tortillas: Arrange the tortillas in a single layer on the prepared baking sheet, and lightly brush each side with a little olive oil. Bake for 5 minutes, or until crisp. Flip the tortillas, and bake for another 5 minutes. Tortillas should be crisp and brown. Remove from the oven and set aside.

Make the smashed black beans: In a small bowl, combine the black beans and half the salsa, smashing the beans until they are slightly creamy and smooth. The objective is to get them spreadable, almost like the consistency of refried beans. You may also use a food processor to achieve a smoother consistency. Add salt and pepper to taste, and set aside.

Mix the crema: In a small bowl, mix the Vegenaise with lime juice to taste. For a slightly thinner consistency, add 1 tablespoon water (or better yet, the reserved jalapeño juice) to taste. Add salt and pepper to taste. Set aside or in the fridge to chill before serving.

Plate the dish: On a plate, arrange 2 or 3 tortillas. Slather tortillas with smashed black beans. Top with a spoonful of walnut chorizo. Drizzle with crema. Garnish with remaining salsa, pickled jalapeños, lettuce, radish, and diced onion. Do a happy dance.

CLEAN-UP NOTES

[S] Lime peel: for Infused Cleaning Vinegar

[S] Garlic, jalapeño, onion skins and tops: for Scrap-Happy Broth

[C] Lettuce and radish scraps, parchment paper (if unwaxed)

[RP] Black beans can, salsa jar, Vegenaise jar: clean and repurpose like a boss.

[RC] / [RP] Tortilla packaging: If it's paper, recycle! If not, repurpose as a storage bag.

ASIAN HOT POT

Savory, brothy goodness for when you want
a big ol' bowl of nourishment

A bad breakup. The flu. A commute in subzero temperatures. Life's woes can often be cured with a piping hot bowl of brothy probiotic goodness. This soup is like a perfectly timed hug from that awesome friend who smells like vanilla candles and recommends the best self-help books. It delivers on flavor without being (1) fussy to make or (2) a caloric shit show. Plus, it's a great way to pack tons of filling, fiber-rich veggies and probiotics (thanks, Miso!) into every delectable bite—erm, slurp.

--- *Makes 2 servings* ---

Prep time: 25 minutes

INGREDIENTS

4 ounces vermicelli rice noodles

1 tablespoon sesame oil, divided

4 ounces fresh shiitake mushrooms, halved

3–4 cups Scrap-Happy Broth or other vegetable broth

½ cup soy sauce, to taste

1 tablespoon minced ginger

1 tablespoon sambal, to taste

4 green onions, sliced on the bias

1½ cups green beans, stems removed

2 carrots, peeled and sliced into thin rounds

3–4 tablespoons white miso, to taste

Prepare the vermicelli: Rice vermicelli noodles are amazingly convenient: they just need to be soaked in hot water and they're ready to go. Bring a medium pot of water to a boil, remove the pot from the heat, and add the noodles. Let the noodles soak until they're tender, about 5 minutes. Drain, pat dry, and cut them into 3-inch lengths.

Make the broth: Heat 1 teaspoon of the sesame oil in a large saucepan over medium-high heat. Add the mushrooms, and cook, stirring occasionally, for

2 minutes. Prepare for your kitchen to smell incredible (sesame oil + mush-rooms = heaven). Add the broth, soy sauce (to taste), ginger (reserving a bit for garnish), and sambal to taste (things can get spicy), and bring to a boil.

Finish the broth: Add the onions and carrots (reserving a small amount of each for garnish), and green beans. Lower the heat, and simmer until the veg-etables are tender, about 6 to 7 minutes. At the very end, add the miso, and stir gently until dissolved (adding last and at a lower heat preserves its probi-otic radness). Add salt and pepper to taste.

Plate the dish: Divide the noodles evenly into bowls. Stir and ladle the broth over the noodles, ensuring each bowl gets lots of mushrooms, green beans, and carrots. Garnish with the remaining green onions and carrots and drizzle with the remaining 2 teaspoons of sesame oil.

CLEAN-UP NOTES

[S] Green bean, carrot, green onion scraps: for Scrap-Happy Broth

AWESOME AVOCADO ALFREDO

With pasta gorgeousness this good, you won't even miss the dairy

South American legend purports that a princess ate the first avocado, and it possessed magical powers. Anyone who's eaten an avocado (so, everyone, I hope?!) would not disagree that this is basically what happens always. This dish is for when you want creamy pasta goodness to jump on lickety-split. Bright basil, juicy tomatoes, and sunny lemon make this the perfect summer pasta, best enjoyed al fresco, listening to the breeze stirring the treetops, getting wine drunk, and watching lightning bugs zip by. It's also really delish cold, which makes it a great next-day lunch.

--- *Makes 2 servings* ---

Total time: 30 minutes

INGREDIENTS

1 large ripe avocado, halved and pitted

1 clove garlic, minced, divided

1 tablespoon lemon juice

1 tablespoon soy sauce

Salt and pepper, to taste

1 tablespoon olive oil

1 green onion, stems removed, thinly sliced on bias

20–30 mini plum or grape tomatoes
(depending on how much you dig tomatoes), halved

½ teaspoon red-pepper flakes

8 ounces preferred pasta (like spaghetti or fettucine)

3 basil sprigs, leaves removed and cut in chiffonade, divided

Make the sauce: Scoop out the avocado, and combine it with half the garlic in a food processor until smooth (if you don't have one, a bowl and a fork or potato masher will do the trick). Add the lemon juice and soy sauce. Season with freshly cracked black pepper to taste.

Blister the tomatoes: Warm a medium pan over medium heat. When hot, add the olive oil and remaining minced garlic. Cook for 30 seconds, or until aromatic, then add the green onion, tomatoes, and half the red-pepper flakes to taste. (Careful on the red pepper. The oil releases its spice, so add according to what your taste buds can handle.) Cook for approximately 7 minutes, or until the tomatoes become blistered and slightly softened. Set aside.

Cook the pasta: Add the pasta to a pot of boiling salted water, and cook for 6 to 8 minutes, or until it is al dente (Italian for "to the tooth," so it still has a little firmness to it); drain.

Assemble the dish: Add the avocado mixture and two-thirds of the basil (reserving remaining for garnish) to the pasta, and toss to combine (tongs work well for this). If desired, add 1 more teaspoon olive oil to the pasta for extra richness. Place a portion of pasta into a shallow dish. Top with a serving of blistered tomatoes, and garnish with remaining basil, any remaining red-pepper flakes, to taste, a pinch of salt, and a crack of fresh black pepper.

CLEAN-UP NOTES

[S] Garlic, basil, and green onion scraps: for Scrap-Happy Broth.

[S] Lemon: for Infused Cleaning Vinegar

[C] Avocado skin and pit

ALMOND JOY

What is pasta without a sprinkle of something umami-laden and lip-smackin' to take things up a notch? Well, here's an almond-based Parmesan to make your less-dairy life way more rad. Best of all, it's easy as hell to make.

Makes 10–15 servings

Total time: 5 minutes

⅓ cup raw almonds

¼ cup nutritional yeast

¼ teaspoon garlic powder

¼ teaspoon salt, or more to taste

Put all the ingredients in a food processor, and pulse until a grated Parmesan-like consistency is achieved. Keep for up to 2 weeks in the fridge. Sprinkle on all the things.

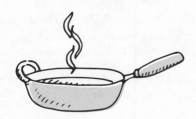

COMFY COZY CHILI

Like a giant warm hug from a smoking-hot dude
after you've hiked through a very magical forest

Rainy days. Snowy days. Days when a hungry soccer team pops over unannounced (does this actually happen?). Sometimes you just need a stick-to-your-ribs meal that involves as much effort as putting a bunch of ingredients in a pot. And here it is! This chili is rich, savory, and tastes like it spent all day simmering, even though it takes only 45 minutes to make (we're using canned beans here, but if you want to use dry, knock yourself out). So prep this bad boy, go watch a show, and return to a bubbling cauldron of dreamy, warming deliciousness. I highly recommend pairing this with a crusty loaf of bread and a good glass of Pinot Noir.

Makes 3 servings

Prep time: 10 minutes
Total time: 45 minutes

INGREDIENTS

1 yellow onion, finely diced

1 teaspoon olive oil

4 ounces cremini mushrooms, diced

2 tablespoons sundried tomatoes, roughly chopped
into thin slivers

1 cup water, or more as desired

1 cup Scrap-Happy Broth or other vegetable broth

5 tablespoons tomato paste

1 (15.5-ounce) can kidney beans

1 tablespoon ground cumin

1 teaspoon garlic powder

1 tablespoon chili powder, or more to taste

2 tablespoons soy sauce

Salt and pepper, to taste

5 parsley sprigs, roughly chopped

Sauté the vegetables: In a stockpot, sauté the onion in the oil for 1 minute, or until it becomes slightly translucent. Add the mushrooms and tomatoes, and sauté until softened, about 5 minutes.

Finish the chili: Stir in the water, broth, tomato paste, beans (including juice from the can), cumin, garlic powder, and chili powder. Bring the chili to a boil, and reduce the heat to low. Let the chili simmer for 20 minutes, or until it thickens to a hearty consistency. Add the soy sauce, salt, and pepper to taste.

Plate the dish: Ladle into bowls, and garnish with fresh parsley. Slip on some comfy socks and your fave TV show, and prepare to slurp your way to coziness.

CLEAN-UP NOTES

[S] Parsley stems, onion scraps, any mushroom scraps: for Scrap-Happy Broth

[RP] Kidney bean can: for a cool craft or planter

BABELY BÁNH MÌ SANDWICHES

Because sometimes you just need a really good sammich

I'm addicted to bánh mì. And because the Vietnamese restaurant by my apartment kept closing due to mysteriously recurring "water issues," I had to create this recipe to basically survive the winter. It's got all of that savory tofu and pickled veggie goodness sandwiched between French bread and slathered with sriracha aioli. Plus, you get to flash pickle your own veggies, the extra of which you'll want to put on everything (except for cereal). Make ahead and wrap in paper for an enviable lunch or picnic take-along.

— *Makes 2 servings* —

Total time: 35 minutes

INGREDIENTS

3 tablespoons Vegenaise

2 tablespoons sriracha, or more to taste, divided

Salt and pepper, to taste

½ cup soy sauce, divided

2 cloves garlic, minced

1 block extra-firm tofu (about 16 ounces),
drained, sliced into ½-inch-thick playing card–sized fillets

2 demi baguettes

1 red onion, finely julienned

2 radishes, sliced into very thin (nearly transparent) rounds

1 jalapeño, thinly sliced (keep the seeds if you want extra heat)

½ cup purple and green cabbage, thinly shredded

1½ cups rice vinegar

¼ cup agave nectar

1 tablespoon olive oil

Optional: 5 sprigs cilantro, roughly chopped

Make the sriracha aioli: In a small bowl, combine the Vegenaise and 1 teaspoon of the sriracha to taste. Stir until the mixture is smooth, and season with salt and pepper to taste. Let it chill in the refrigerator until it is ready to serve.

Marinate the tofu: In another bowl, combine half the soy sauce and all the garlic. Cover the tofu fillets with the mixture in a glass container, and let them marinate for 5 minutes, then remove; reserve the marinade.

Toast the bread: If desired, warm your baguettes in the oven until desired softness or crustiness is reached. Slice the baguettes in half lengthwise, and keep them warm until ready to serve.

Pickle the veggies: In a bowl, combine the onion, radish, jalapeño, and cabbage, as you will be pickling these.

In a large saucepan, combine the vinegar and remaining soy sauce over high heat. Once boiling slightly (after about 3 minutes), stir in the agave and half the remaining sriracha. Remove from heat, and allow to cool for 3 minutes. Pour the liquid over the onion, radish, jalapeño, and cabbage, ensuring they are covered completely with the vinegar mixture. Add salt and pepper to taste. Place in the refrigerator or freezer for 15 minutes to cool.

Cook the tofu: While the veggies cool, heat a skillet on high and add the olive oil. Place the marinated tofu fillets in the skillet, and cook until they're browned on each side, about 5 to 7 minutes. If the fillets get a little dry, pour some of the reserved marinade over them as they cook. Once they have reached your desired char, flip and repeat on the other side. Remove the fillets from the skillet, and allow them to cool on a plate.

Plate the dish: On plates—or, for a fun street food–style touch, atop parchment paper—assemble your sandwiches. Slather the aioli on the bottom half of the baguette. Add the tofu fillets, and cover with slightly drained pickled veggies (but keep the liquid for future pickling). Slather more sriracha aioli on the top of the baguette and top with fresh chopped cilantro if you're one of those people who like cilantro (I'm not). Add remaining sriracha to punch up the experience. Try not to eat both sandwiches in one sitting (points to self).

CLEAN-UP NOTES

[S] Cabbage, onion, jalapeño, cilantro, and garlic scraps: for Scrap-Happy Broth

[S] Pickling liquid: for future pickling adventures or to add to olive oil and lemon for a sassy salad dressing

[C] Radish scraps

[RC] Tofu packaging, if recyclable

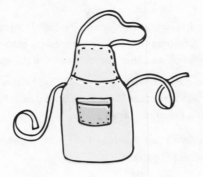

Puttin' on the Ritz (aka Fancier Fare)

Oh, you fancy, huh? Sometimes life calls for LBDs over boyfriend jeans and stilettos over sensible flats. And when those occasions pop on your calendar, you'll be prepared with this culinary closet full of recipes that dazzle like a lethal cocktail of sequins, Spanx, and push-up bras.

QUINOA-STUFFED ACORN SQUASH

Sometimes holidays happen.
And when they do, these little bowls of
deliciousness have your back.

Times of celebration can cause the most anxiety among the plant-powered crowd. Why? Because for every amazing, inquisitive, kind friend or relative who supports your shift to a cruelty-free diet, there will be at least one dickhead who tries to sneak you sausage or ply you with bacon. Moreover, many people will not know how to feed a vegetarian or vegan, and thus, you may be stuck with a sad Thanksgiving meal consisting of dinner rolls and dry romaine lettuce. Make things easy for any host, and avoid the problem altogether by BYOing the veggie goodness, and make this your go-to take-along for those tense holiday gatherings and potlucks. It's a satisfying enough main for you (and anyone else, carnivores included), and it serves as a lovely complement to the meatier fare your relatives may be enjoying without looking like you're trying to compete with whatever the host is making. That said, this is going to be the best thing on the table, so try not to be too smug about it, okay? Cool.

———————————— *Makes 4 servings* ————————————

Prep time: 20 minutes
Total time: 45 minutes

INGREDIENTS

2 acorn squash, halved and seeded,
with a bit cut off bottom so it can lay flat

2 tablespoons olive oil, divided

Salt and pepper, to taste

1½ cups water, lightly salted

1¼ cups quinoa (I like tricolor)

1 cup Scrap-Happy Broth or other vegetable broth

1 yellow onion, finely diced

2 cloves garlic, minced

½ cup raw pecans

¼ cup dried cranberries

2 thyme sprigs, leaves pulled from stems

½ cup white cooking wine

¼ cup maple syrup

Preheat the oven to 400°F, and prepare a baking sheet with parchment or foil.

Roast the acorn squash: Brush the orange innards of the squash halves with 1 tablespoon oil and add a dash of salt and pepper. Place the four squash halves open-side-down on the baking sheet, and roast for 25 minutes, or until the meat is tender and slightly browned.

Cook the quinoa: While the squash is roasting, bring the salted water, quinoa, and broth to a boil. Once boiling, reduce heat to low, and simmer for 10 minutes, or until all the water is absorbed. Remove the quinoa from heat, salt and pepper to taste, fluff with a fork, and set aside.

Prepare the quinoa stuffing: While the quinoa is cooking, in a skillet, sauté 1 tablespoon olive oil, the onion, and garlic together until they are translucent, about 3 minutes. Add the pecans, and sauté for another 2 minutes. Then stir in the cooked quinoa, cranberries, thyme (reserving a pinch for garnish), and white wine. Salt and pepper to taste, remove from heat, and set aside until you are ready to stuff the squash.

Stuff and roast the squash: Remove the squash from the oven, and flip open-side-up. Add ½ cup or more of the quinoa mixture to the hollow of each squash half. Place them back in the oven for 10 to 12 minutes, or until the quinoa is slightly crisp and the squash has caramelized.

Place a stuffed acorn squash on each plate. Garnish with remaining thyme and a light drizzle of maple syrup. Add salt and pepper to taste.

CLEAN-UP NOTES

[S] Onion, garlic, thyme scraps: for Scrap-Happy Broth

[C] Squash skins and seeds, parchment paper (if unwaxed)

BBQ TOFU TACOS

A fiesta in your mouth, but not a party in your pants.
Best tacos ever.

If you're Texan like me, sometimes you want tacos and sometimes you want BBQ. And boy howdy, do these tacos answer the call like none other. They're also really fucking simple, which is grand because I'm usually drunk when this blessed craving strikes. These are also great for serving to people who think that tofu is disgusting, because they're meaty and flavorful. As your mom always said, if someone has nothing nice to say, stuff a taco in their mouth and problem solved.

Makes 2 servings, 6 tacos

Total time: 25 minutes

INGREDIENTS

3 green onion stems, finely diced

3 cups purple cabbage, finely shredded

½ cup Annie's Goddess Dressing
(or TJ's Goddess Dressing)

1 lime, juiced

Salt and pepper, to taste

1 tablespoon olive oil

1 package (about 14 ounces) extra-firm tofu,
drained and diced into ¼-inch pieces

1 teaspoon cumin

½ teaspoon smoked paprika

½ teaspoon ground ginger

½ cup vegan BBQ sauce

⅛ cup water, if needed

1 package corn tortillas (about 6)

Optional: 5 sprigs cilantro, roughly chopped

Make the slaw: In a medium bowl, combine the green onion, cabbage, goddess dressing, and lime juice. Add salt and pepper to taste. Place covered in refrigerator to chill before serving.

Prepare the tofu: Heat a skillet over medium-high heat, then add the olive oil and diced tofu. Add the cumin, smoked paprika, and ground ginger. Stir to coat the tofu, and cook until tofu becomes aromatic and slightly browned, about 8 minutes.

Once cooked, reduce heat to low-medium and add BBQ sauce (and water, if you desire a thinner consistency). Coat tofu completely and cook for another 5 minutes. Remove from heat.

Warm tortillas: Cover tortillas in a paper towel and microwave for about 1 minute or until supple. Alternatively, you can warm tortillas directly on a stove burner at low heat (this is not for folks who don't like to monitor their food) until soft. Whatever floats your boat, peeps.

Assemble your tacos: Place 3 tortillas on a plate, add the tofu mixture, and top with chilled slaw and freshly chopped cilantro, if desired. Enjoy with a margarita and nice people.

CLEAN-UP NOTES

[S] Green onion, cilantro, and cabbage scraps: for Scrap-Happy Broth

[RC] / [RP] Tortilla packaging: If paper, recycle! If not, consider reusing.

[S] Lime: For Infused Cleaning Vinegar.

NONNA'S TRUFFLED MUSHROOM RISOTTO

A culinary visit to Florence, minus the pricey plane ticket

My grandmother is from Northern Italy. She's also 106 years old and says cool stuff like "What do I care what day it is?" or "My God, Ashlee, you drive like a man!" I made this recipe in homage to her, because risotto is the crown jewel of Northern Italian cooking. Gussy up this date-night staple by adding aphrodisiacal wild mushrooms and sinful truffle oil. Much like a good love affair, preparing authentic risotto requires undivided attention, so be sure to have a solid 15 to 20 minutes to devote to deglazing and stirring, deglazing and stirring. The reward will be worth the effort. This is also an excellent recipe for those undrunk bottles of white wine kicking around your home. (Shyeah right, like that's something I have.)

Makes 2 servings

Total time: 50 minutes

INGREDIENTS

2 teaspoons olive oil, divided

8 ounces fresh wild mushrooms (can also be a mix of button, shiitake, and cremini mushrooms), finely chopped

1 shallot, finely diced

1 cup Arborio rice

¼ cup white cooking wine

4 cups Scrap-Happy Broth, or any vegetable broth, warmed

2 tablespoons vegan butter

6 chives, halved and finely diced, with 1 stalk reserved for garnish

3 tablespoons nutritional yeast

Salt, to taste

½ teaspoon crushed peppercorns

3 parsley sprigs, finely chopped

2 teaspoons truffle oil

Sauté the mushrooms: In a skillet, warm 1 teaspoon olive oil and the mushrooms over medium-high heat. Once the mushrooms are aromatic and slightly caramelized (about 5 minutes), remove from heat and transfer to a dish.

Start the risotto: In the same skillet used to cook the mushrooms, add 1 teaspoon olive oil and the shallot, and cook over medium heat for 1 to 2 minutes, or until aromatic. Stir in the rice, coating with the oil and shallot. After about 2 minutes, when the rice has become a bit translucent, pour in the white wine, stirring constantly until it is fully absorbed and the alcohol has been cooked off.

Stir the risotto: Reduce heat to low-medium, add ½ cup warmed broth (straining the mushrooms and leaving them in the broth pan) to the rice, and stir until the broth is absorbed; continue adding broth ½ cup at a time (this is called *cottura* in Italian) whenever the pan seems to be getting dry. (My grandmother always recommended singing a song that lasts a few minutes. When it's over, that's when you know to add more liquid.) Stir constantly until the liquid is absorbed and the rice becomes tender, about 20 to 25 minutes. The sauce should be silky and the rice chewy but not crunchy. If the risotto has not yet reached this texture after 25 minutes, add more broth little by little, and continue the process until you achieve your desired texture (taking little bites at a time).

Finish the risotto: Once the risotto is tender, remove from heat, and stir in any remaining broth, the sautéed mushrooms, vegan butter, diced chives (reserving remaining stalk for garnish), nutritional yeast, and salt and freshly crushed peppercorns to taste.

Plate the dish: Ladle a serving of risotto onto a plate or into shallow dish. Garnish with halved chive stalk, parsley, any remaining crushed peppercorns to taste, and a luxurious drizzle of truffle oil.

CLEAN-UP NOTES

[S] Shallot scraps, chive and parsley stems, mushroom scraps:
for Scrap-Happy Broth

STEAK HOUSE SERENADE

Stick-to-your ribs, fork-and-knife meal
that doesn't use anyone's ribs

You may think that eating plant-based means the end of your dalliances with steak houses. This simply isn't true (there are lots of things you can get at a steak house, friend), but for an at-home experience, this meal really conjures up the flavors and aromas of a meaty meal. It's perfect for when you're trying to impress (but don't want to look like you're trying, like, homemade macarons hard), especially finicky eaters (or people who think vegan food is weird). A juicy, umami-laden portobello mushroom steak sits atop fluffy garlic mashed potatoes and is crowned with savory, smooth mushroom gravy. Pair with a "nice green vegetable," as my mother would say, a solid glass of Pinot Noir, and maybe some cloth napkins to give that home-cooked-but-fancy-as-fuck vibe, and prepare for people to actually offer to do the dishes or run you a bubble bath.

— *Makes 2 servings* —
Prep time: 20 minutes
Total time: 40 minutes

INGREDIENTS

FOR THE MUSHROOMS:
4 portobello mushrooms (stems and caps)

3 tablespoons balsamic vinegar

3 tablespoons olive oil

1 tablespoon soy sauce

½ teaspoon dried oregano

2 cloves garlic

Salt and pepper, to taste

FOR THE POTATOES:

12 ounces Yukon Gold potatoes
(about 6–7 depending on size), skin on

3 cloves garlic, peeled

¼ cup vegan butter, divided

¼ teaspoon salt

Pepper, to taste

3 chives, finely diced

FOR THE GRAVY:

1 teaspoon olive oil

½ cup finely diced yellow onion

¾ cup finely diced cremini mushrooms
(plus the stems from the Portobello caps)

¼ cup all-purpose flour

4 cups Scrap-Happy Broth

1 teaspoon soy sauce

Salt and pepper, to taste

FOR THE MUSHROOMS:

Clean the portobello mushrooms: Remove the stems (reserve them for the gravy) and lightly scrub them under cold water to remove any dirt. Pat dry and place in a shallow glass baking dish.

Make the marinade: In a small bowl, whisk together the balsamic vinegar, olive oil, soy sauce, oregano, and a pinch of salt and pepper. Pour the marinade on each cap, using your fingers to ensure they're totally coated. Allow to marinate for at least 10 minutes (these can marinate all day in the fridge, though, if you prefer).

Once marinated and about 15 minutes before desired serving time, lightly grease a skillet or grill pan and set on the stove over medium-high heat.

Cook the mushrooms: Once the pan is warm, add the mushroom caps and cook for about 6 to 10 minutes on each side, until the edges of the caps become slightly wilted and, if using a grill pan, nice grill mark indentations form. Brush any extra marinade on them as they cook.

FOR THE POTATOES:

Cook the potatoes and garlic: Peel and cut potatoes into 2-inch cubes. Add the potatoes and peeled garlic cloves to a medium pot, cover with water, salt lightly, and bring to a boil. Reduce to a simmer and cook until you can easily poke the potatoes with a fork, 16 to 20 minutes. Reserve ¼ cup cooking liquid. Strain potatoes and garlic in a colander and return to pot.

Make the mash: Add half the vegan butter, the salt, and a pinch of pepper and mash until smooth. If necessary, add reserved cooking liquid and 1 tablespoon remaining vegan butter at a time until desired consistency is reached.

FOR THE GRAVY:

In a large skillet over medium-high heat, heat 1 teaspoon of olive oil and sauté the diced onion and mushrooms, stirring occasionally. Intermittently add a sprinkle of the flour and ½ cup of vegetable broth at a time, stirring in as you go, until the gravy has thickened (use less flour if you prefer a thinner gravy) and the mushroom stems are slightly browned, about 8 to 10 minutes. Add soy sauce and salt and pepper to taste.

Tip: The gravy is good to go as it is, but for a cream gravy, you can add the entire mixture to a blender (or use an immersion blender) and puree until smooth. Or, for a smoother gravy with no mushroom bits, you can pass thru a mesh strainer.

Plate the dish: Add a generous dollop of mashed potatoes to two plates. Top with any remaining vegan butter and chives if desired, and add salt and pepper to taste. Nestle two portobello steaks atop the mashed potatoes. Serve with gravy on the side, or drizzle gravy atop the entire dish. Eat the fuck up.

CLEAN-UP NOTES

[S] Garlic and onion skins, chive scraps, mushroom scraps:
for Scrap-Happy Broth

P.M.S., S.O.S.
(aka Sweet Thangs)

JAMOCHA SILK PIE

Creamy, sweet, coffee-ish, perfect.
Oh, and did I mention no-bake? YASSSSS.

I have a confession to make: as a young girl growing up in Texas, one of my favorite things to do was to roll down to the Arby's on a hot day and get a cool, creamy jamocha shake. Man, that shit was good. A few times in life you get lucky and become an instant genius. At least, that's what happened to me when I blended (pun totally intended) my nostalgic crush on shitty, now-verboten fast-food milk shakes with my near-disturbing love for pie. Now, this is not a health food, BUT it is way more sensible than your average French silk–style pie, which is traditionally made with gobs of cream, and it's just as delish. Topped with my go-to Whip It Good "Cream" (page 170), this shit is TDF.

Makes 8 servings (or 1, if you're me)

Prep time: 10 minutes
Total time: 1 hour 15 minutes
(most of which is just the pie chilling)

INGREDIENTS

1 (16-ounce) block silken tofu, drained
(the squidgy kind of tofu)

2 tablespoons cocoa powder

1 teaspoon vanilla extract

¼–½ cup brewed coffee or espresso, divided

1 cup unsweetened, flaked coconut, divided

1 cup vegan dark or bittersweet chocolate chips

2 tablespoons maple syrup, to taste

Pinch of salt

½ cup chopped, toasted pecans, divided

1 honey-free vegan graham cracker crust
(or make your own, or go crustless)

Optional: Whip It Good "Cream" (page 170) for topping

Prepare the filling: In a blender, combine the tofu, cocoa powder, vanilla, coffee (reserving 1 tablespoon for the chocolate mixture in Step 2), and ⅔ cup of the coconut; blend until smooth.

Melt the chocolate: In a double boiler or microwave-safe bowl, combine the chocolate chips and remaining coffee; melt and stir until smooth. Remove from heat and allow to cool for a few minutes, and then add to the tofu mixture in the blender.

Finish the filling: Blend the mixture together again, and taste. Add a pinch of salt and additional maple syrup if desired. I prefer my pie a bit on the rich and bittersweet side (which pairs so nicely with gobs of whipped coconut cream or aquafaba whip), but hey, to each her own.

Assemble the pie: Once the mixture is smooth, transfer it to a bowl and manually stir in the pecans (don't blend in with your blender or the pie will take on a bitter taste) and remaining coconut flakes. Pour the batter into the prepared pie crust; cover and place in the freezer for 30 minutes or in the refrigerator overnight to firm up.

Optional: If you don't dig on pie crust, pour the filling into glasses, layer with nondairy whip, pecans, and coconut, and, by god, firm them up and enjoy them as rich, dreamy parfaits.

Serve and store: Once the pie reaches your desired firmness, cut into eight equal pieces (or a few massive pieces), and crown with your whip of choice and garnish with more toasted pecans and coconut.

This pie will keep well for 4 days when covered and stored in the fridge. There is absolutely no way, however, that you won't eat it before then.

CLEAN-UP NOTES

[RC] / [RP] Tofu packaging, pie crust pan
(if you used a store-bought crust in an aluminum pan)

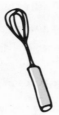

WHIP IT GOOD "CREAM"

Listen, I am no pie snob. I'll eat pretty much any and all pie if offered to me. That said, I also know the universal truth that all pie is better with criminal amounts of creamy, vanilla-y whipped topping. And luckily, you've got just the stuff kicking around, masquerading as something you'd normally let go to waste down the drain, in your kitchen. This whip uses aquafaba, the liquid from canned chickpeas, and it actually makes a totally convincing, pillowy, dreamy whipped topping for this pie (and any other pie you dream up).

Makes 2 cups

Total time: 15 minutes

INGREDIENTS:

Liquid from 1 (15-ounce) can of chickpeas
(aka aquafaba), drained and reserved

⅛ teaspoon cream of tartar

1 teaspoon vanilla extract
(or, the seeds from ½ vanilla bean)

2 tablespoons superfine sugar

In a bowl (allow for space because this mixture is gonna get whipped, guys) or a blender with a whipping blade, add the aquafaba, cream of tartar, and vanilla extract or seeds. If using a hand- or standing blender, put beaters on whipping mode and slowly add the sugar until mixture goes from frothy to fluffy, about 15 minutes. If using the blender with whipping blade, add the sugar once the mixture begins to go from frothy to forming peaks. Keep chilled and use immediately to crown all the desserts (and random lovers who come over).

TUESDAY'S COOKIE

*If chocolate chip cookies and peanut butter
got hitched and honeymooned in Hawaii*

When I first became vegan, I got way into baking, which is weird because I'm too rebellious to follow recipes and baking kind of hinges on precision. Always in search of new cookie combos, I instituted something called "Tuesday's Cookie" on my blog—kicked off by this happy accident recipe—in which I'd post a new cookie recipe every Tuesday. The concept didn't last until the water got hot, because I was a terribly negligent blogger, but this recipe was such a hit that I *still* get fan letters about it. If you like chocolate, peanut butter, and coconut, well, you'll probably really like these. This also makes a dope cookie dough to take big bites from whenever. Just sharing the trade secrets, guys.

Makes about 18 cookies

Prep time: 10 minutes
Total time: 25 minutes

INGREDIENTS

1½ cups all-purpose flour

½ cup sugar

½ cup brown sugar, packed

½ teaspoon baking soda

¾ teaspoon baking powder

1 teaspoon salt

⅓ cup unrefined coconut oil

1 teaspoon vanilla extract

½ cup creamy peanut butter (I use homemade
and feel it makes the dough easier to work with
and imparts a richer flavor)

¼ cup White Witch Almond Milk, or other almond milk

½ cup unsweetened flaked coconut

½ cup vegan dark chocolate chips

Preheat oven to 375°F (yes, certain recipes call for preheating for optimal results and this is one of 'em), and prepare two baking sheets with Silpat liners or parchment paper.

Mix the dry ingredients: In a large mixing bowl, sift the flour, sugars, baking soda, baking powder, and salt together.

Mix the wet ingredients: In a separate bowl, melt the coconut oil in a double boiler or the microwave. Once it's melted, stir in the vanilla and peanut butter. Add the oil mixture to the larger bowl's dry mixture; stir until it is slightly assimilated.

Create the dough: One by one, fold in the coconut and chocolate chips, followed by even portions of the almond milk as you go to enable easier mixing. Mix until the dough is firm enough to work with and the chips and coconut flakes are distributed throughout the dough.

Roll and bake: Using your hands, roll the dough into 1¼-inch balls, spacing them out on the prepared baking sheets. Bake at 375°F for 11 to 15 minutes, pressing down lightly on the cookies midway thru baking—11 minutes for a softer cookie (my personal favorite), 15 for a firmer cookie. Remove from oven and allow to fully cool on the baking sheet or a cookie rack so they firm up in the center.

HOT TIP: If you're leaving the dough as cookie dough, it can easily be frozen for up to 2 weeks (perfect for grabbing, unwrapping, and taking giant bites out of when you want to eat your feelings). When you're ready to bake, just defrost and follow the baking instructions.

CLEAN-UP NOTES

[C] Parchment paper (if unwaxed)

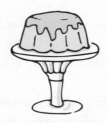

KOOL & THE GANG CAKE

Celebrate good times . . . with this cake

Hey, we're all coexisting on this spinning planet, and that's pretty crazy, huh? We inhale oxygen wihout having to think about it. You're able to see and read and touch this book. Thesis: Life is worth celebrating. So for all the birthdays, congrats, showers, anniversaries, and PTA-pressured bake sales, I turn to this simple-but-celebratory vanilla cake (which can easily be converted into cupcakes). It's like the Helmut Lang black blazer I scored at a thrift store last year—easily dressed up or down and perfect for all occasions.

Makes 24 cupcakes; one 8-inch, 3-layer cake;
——— one 12-inch, 2-layer cake; or 1 enormous 24-inch sheet cake ———

Prep time: 12 minutes
Total time: 40 minutes

INGREDIENTS

FOR THE CAKE

2 cups White Witch Almond Milk, or other almond milk

1 tablespoon fresh lemon juice

3 cups unbleached all-purpose flour

1½ cups sugar

1 tablespoon baking powder

1 teaspoon baking soda

1 teaspoon salt

¾ cup unrefined coconut oil, melted

4½ teaspoons vanilla extract

FOR THE BUTTERCREAM FROSTING

TIP: If you're making a layered cake,
double this frosting recipe

½ cup vegan butter, softened

½ cup vegan shortening, softened

4 cups powdered sugar

1 teaspoon vanilla extract,
or the seeds of 1 vanilla bean (my preference)

¼ cup White Witch Almond Milk
or other unsweetened nut milk, or more as needed

TO GARNISH (OPTIONAL)

Fresh raspberries or strawberries

Coconut flakes

Preheat oven to 350°F. Prepare your cake pan(s) or muffin tins by coating them with coconut oil and/or adding cupcake sleeves if making cupcakes.

Create "buttermilk": In a small bowl, combine the milk and lemon juice. Let stand for 2 minutes.

Combine dry ingredients: In a separate large bowl, combine the flour, sugar, baking powder, baking soda, and salt.

Make the batter and bake: Slowly add the coconut oil, vanilla, and "buttermilk" to the dry ingredients, being careful to not overstir. Once mixed, pour or spoon the batter into the cake or muffin pans, and bake for 20 minutes for cupcakes and 25 to 30 minutes for cakes, or until the center is set and a toothpick comes out cleanly with just a few crumbs.

Make the frosting: While the cake is baking, cream together the vegan butter and shortening in a stand mixer or with a hand mixer until fluffy. While beaters are still going, slowly add in powdered sugar 1 cup at a time until completely assimilated. Add in vanilla extract (or vanilla beans) and almond milk, and mix on high for 5 minutes until all ingredients are creamed together and frosting is dense and fluffy.

Cool and frost: After removing the cake or cupcakes from the oven, allow them to cool for a few minutes in the pan(s) (a cooling rack is really ace for this). Remove from the pans and allow them to cool completely before frosting (frosting a warm cake is a fucking nightmare). Use a spatula or icing knife to evenly distribute the frosting. If desired, garnish the cake with fresh raspberries, strawberries, or coconut flakes. Serve immediately, and store extras covered, at room temperature, for up to 3 days.

CLEAN-UP NOTES

[S] Lemon: for Infused Cleaning Vinegar

[C] Vanilla pod

QUICK HITS
IN THE KITCHEN

Few things will make a dent in environmental degradation like changing the way you eat and shop for food. Here are some wham-bam-thank-you-ma'am! fast tips that'll have you helping our planetary pal in five minutes or less.

- *Enjoy one (or more) vegan meal today. And then another one tomorrow. And another one. And another one. You'll soon become the DJ Khaled of your daily diet.*

- *Find a dope veggie restaurant in your hood, and make a plan to visit with your posse, an open mind, and a grumbling tum.*

- *Build a reusable kit for grocery shopping from secondhand jars, upcycled cloth bags, and reusable totes. Now put it wherever you will see it and use it, like your car if you drive to the store or your entryway.*

- *Research bulk bin options in your area. The Zero Waste Home Bulk Finder is a great place to start, as are local forums and groups dedicated to zero-waste living. Find them, love them, and then set a date to check these places out and feast your eyes on their bounty of unpackaged bliss.*

- *Find your nearest farmers' market. Sign up for a CSA.*

- *Walk to get your groceries. Then walk home with them. Feel strong like bull.*

- *Start a container in your freezer for saving vegetable scraps. At the end of the week, make my Scrap-Happy Vegetable Broth.*

Give a Shit:

In Your Closet

I t's 7 a.m.: Do you know what you're wearing today? Chances are, you don't. And that's cool. I too like to live dangerously. I am probably also still asleep. Anywho, let's talk about clothes for a sec. They're kind of important. Trends come and go, but one universal truth remains: unless you're living in a nudist colony (in which case, call me), you gotta get dressed every damn day. Sure, you may not always feel like it (hi, election malaise and bad Tinder date), but clothing yourself with confidence is a big part of giving a shit. And to dress for the battle called life, you need to combine style with shit-giving substance.

In the age of fast-fashion sweatshops but also choices like "zero waste" and "upcycled," you have lots of options. And that breadth of choices can be confusing as hell. To further complicate matters, we're also bombarded with stealthy marketing that paints shopping as the salve for all our problems. Feeling sad? Get a new shirt! Hot date? Buy four pairs of shoes "just in case." And we are suckers for it because, well, we're human. And yet constant consumption can be one of the most isolating activities on the planet, which is especially detrimental at a time when we need authentic human connection more than ever.

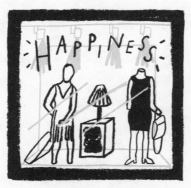

MORE ≠ BETTER

Here's my theory on what and why we buy: Picture a crummy day at work. You bust out of those doors, whispering, "Go pound sand, Todd," under your breath and make your way to the mall, where the siren song of impossibly small mannequins clad in the latest glittering ensembles brings you an odd, much-needed sense of comfort. Sure, boss-man Todd won't care that you've just spent $132.90 on some crap you'll probably never wear, and the beep of your already-stretched-thin credit card being charged gives you mild angina, but you're shopping, dammit! And there's nothing more American or therapeutic than that! Right!? Wrong.

See, those window displays were made for you. Just like magazine and television advertisements, they're designed to entice you with an alternative, unattainable version of reality. One where bosses are amazing, the living's always easy, bodies are flawless, money abounds, and music video dance parties are happening everywhere all the time (I wish). But the truth is that the relief you're seeking is almost never at the stores. Sure, a good bottle of wine or a pretty dress can make you feel like a million bucks . . . temporarily. They're quick fixes. And quick fixes have fiscal, karmic, and ecological tolls. Studies show that 90 percent of our purchasing decisions are not made consciously.[1] Moreover, there's the ever-present battle between utilitarian purchasing ("I need snow boots because it's snowing") and hedonic spending ("That cell phone ad just makes me feel joy!"), further complicating the pursuit of mindful consumption. The emotional dupe here leads us to spend money and feel worse in the long run.

Don't believe me? Consider something as simple as the new arrival schedules at some of the most notorious fast-fashion retailers: H&M and Forever 21 receive daily shipments of new merch, while Topshop introduces four hundred new styles online every single week.[2] Sure, trends change quickly, but this practice isn't about keeping up with trends; it's about creating so many options that no matter how vigilant a shopper you are, you'll always feel inadequate and ill equipped. And because our emotionally based purchases are not well thought out, they're more likely to support the horrors of fast fashion, from sweatshops, child labor, and slavery to environmental degradation and animal cruelty. When we browse from a rational, measured headspace, we're more likely to think twice about buying items that so blatantly support companies that don't give a shit.

WHY THE GARMENT INDUSTRY IS FUCKED UP

Clothes aren't just textiles and patterns; they're physical embodiments of our values. Remember when just a chapter ago I mentioned that animal agriculture is one of the largest contributors to climate change? Well, it seems logical that this chapter follows because, HELLO, the global fashion industry is often heralded as the second-biggest polluter in the world (although some sources say it hovers closer to fourth or fifth—but still not great).[3]

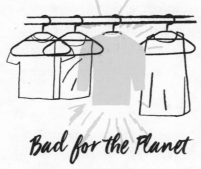

Bad for the Planet

The apparel industry is responsible for 10 percent of all global carbon emissions and is the second-highest polluter of clean water.[4] And that's not all. A report published in *MIT News* found that most fast-fashion retailers outsource their production to developing countries (where cheap resources and labor are plentiful) that often depend on coal power for electricity. The 150 billion pieces produced globally every year require shit-tons of coal power.[5] This is what we'd call a freaking terrible carbon footprint. And because most items aren't sold where they're produced, those garments require loads of nonrenewable oil to get to consumers.

And that's just the ecological toll of fashion manufacturing. When we get to how much waste is created in the end cycle of a garment, you'll want to breathe into a paper bag. You'd think with all these nice, new, resource-hogging wears, we'd cherish them forever, right? Nah. Instead, Americans discard fourteen billion pounds of textiles per year, 85 percent of which end up in landfills.[6] To put that into perspective, that's eighty-two pounds per person, or a collective twenty-one billion pounds tossed away every single year. The EPA estimates that diverting just clothing from landfills would be the eco-equivalent of taking 7.3 million cars and their attendant CO_2 emissions off the road.[7] And that's just clothes! The US Department of Interior approximates that Americans throw away three hundred million pairs of shoes each year, and those suckers take thousands of years to break down in a landfill, emitting serious methane as they embark on their not-so-fantastic voyage to the great beyond.[8]

Bad for People

The garment industry, especially overseas in countries like Bangladesh, China, Vietnam, India, and Indonesia, is a bit like the Wild West, except not in a fun saloon-girl kind of way. Sweatshops are very real, as are the torture, trafficking, slavery, dangerous working conditions, and child labor they encourage and thrive on. Most of what we buy off the rack is implicated because it's pretty much impossible to produce $12 jeans without some collateral damage, usually in the form of women and children who work eighteen-hour days without a freaking bathroom break. The International Labour Organization (ILO) estimates that 168 million children—14 percent of the world's kiddos—are involved in child labor today.[9] How can this be possible, you ask? Children in developing countries, due to a variety of dire circumstances, are more likely to work for low pay in hazardous conditions. And child labor is so widespread that even well-known brands like Adidas, H&M, and Nike have unknowingly used manufacturers exposed for relying on child labor, citing that supply chain networks are so complex that it's virtually "impossible to be in full control."[10] Upon a breaking expose in 2015, these companies, along with others, have since helped workers mobilize to demand better wages and safer conditions.

Moreover, even though the garment sector is composed of 80 percent women, making it the largest employer of females globally, such employment is at the bottom of the hierarchy, and less than 2 percent of those women earn a living wage.[11] This means that most workers can't even afford to buy the garments they produce, let alone provide for their families. If feminism is important to you—as it should be for everyone—a great way to walk the talk is by embracing slower, ethical fashion. And as with any for-profit industry that hinges on the sweat of vulnerable persons, abuse and human rights violations run rampant. Garment workers who attempt to organize, don't produce fast enough, or get pregnant can be abused, sexually harassed, discriminated against, intimidated with threats of harm to their families, and denied pay, water, and restroom breaks.[12] Upon writing this, news broke of ZARA shoppers in Istanbul finding tags on their garments sewn by Turkish workers from the Bravo Tekstil factory saying, "I made this item you are going to buy, but I didn't get paid for it."—a true cry for help from the exploited.[13]

To throw even more fuel onto this tire fire, many workers toil in unsafe, grossly underregulated facilities, huffing illness-causing chemicals and airborne matter. You might remember the 2013 Rana Plaza building collapse in Bangladesh that killed more than eleven hundred and injured over two thousand garment workers. Considered one of fashion's deadliest events to date, this horrific incident could easily have been prevented with facility inspections, regulations, and maintenance. Crumbling factories, oppressive temperatures, abuse, and hours laboring in fields and at machines are par for the course in the garment industry. That $6 T-shirt doesn't seem like such a sweet deal anymore, does it?

Bad for Animals

I'm going to tell you something you already know but don't want to hear: animals don't willingly give us their furs, skins, feathers, and other body parts because they want us to look on trend. Whether procured as slaughterhouse byproducts or from seriously barbaric breed-for-slaughter operations, millions of animals like cows, foxes, sheep, geese, rabbits, dogs, cats, reptiles, and seals suffer and die each year for fashion. And like their exploited agricultural counterparts, the endings aren't always humane. Animals killed for fur and exotic skins are often bludgeoned, anally electrocuted, hanged, drowned, or skinned alive.

Wool, angora, and down aren't cuddly either. Sheep and cashmere goats often live in suffocating heat, are restrained and slashed when sheared, and, after they've exhausted their wool-bearing heyday, are transported to other countries where they either die en route or are slaughtered for food. Shearling is actually sheep's skin with the wool still attached. Karakul, also called broadtail, a material prized by luxury labels like Michael Kors and Givenchy, is the product of slaughtering newborn or in-utero fetal lambs (I don't even need to detail how fucked up that process is). Rabbits and birds are restrained while their fur and feathers are painfully ripped from their bodies with no anesthetic, often leaving them exposed to the elements, bleeding, and in immense pain.

And what about leather? Isn't it actually sort of eco-friendly because it's natural and comes from cows we're eating already anyway? Cute. That's what I used to think too. However, the EPA cites that conventional leather tanning and processing, which is usually a byproduct of animal agriculture, as prime polluter of waterways, and the chemical-laden tanning process (which keeps leather from, ya know, decomposing on us) has not only been cited in certain incidents as being done by children, but is also replete with carcinogens that can sicken workers and surrounding communities.[14]

Even insects aren't immune to fashion brutality: to produce a single pound of silk, three thousand silkworms (which are scientifically proven to have physical responses to pain) are steamed or gassed alive. Who needs a shot right now? (Raises hand.)

HOW NOT TO DRESS LIKE A JERK

I know what you're thinking: "What can I wear now that everything makes me feel like an asshole?!" I hear you, but you needn't go naked. There are loads of affordable, stylin' ethical options that won't make you look like a sister wife. The ills of fast fashion exist solely because consumers (hi, that's you and me) create demand, which means we can easily right this wrong by paring down, refreshing our habits, and pumping the breaks on our purchasing. And because everything starts with reevaluating what's important to us, you know I'm about to wax poetic again about minimizing.

Fewer but Better

Pet rocks, bushy male sideburns, and the phrase "in your face"—the 1970s gave us some pretty remarkable cultural contributions. Chief among them is the badass capsule wardrobe. The concept of a capsule is to curate a small wardrobe composed of timeless essentials (seasonally augmented with some trendier items). Capsule wardrobes have myriad benefits (like always having chic AF shit to wear), but my fave is the fact that they really encourage you to focus on quality over quantity, which helps to reinforce the practice of buying fewer items but with more solid ethical cred.

Here's the skinny: most of us only wear 13 to 20 percent of our closet.[15] Anecdotally, we have a hunch this is true when coworkers remark, "Wow, I feel like you wear that outfit every Thursday." Um, I do. Humans are creatures of habit, and thus, we reach for our favorites—the comfortable, easy pieces that make us feel fab. The rest of your wardrobe looks great on hangers but is usually just collecting dust. Don't believe me? Go about your life for a month, and once you've worn an item, hang it and turn it in the opposite direction. At the end of the month, count how many turned hangers you've got relative to the others and call me so I can say I told you so.

Although the presence of these extra, lesser-worn clothes may seem innocuous, all those extra duds are essentially white noise distracting us from more streamlined, peaceful getting-ready routines. Moreover, the shopping that brought those unused items to your closet in the first place sucks up precious time and money. With a capsule wardrobe, you plan and shop once and no more than that during the season. The Carrie Bradshaws among us may be hyperventilating right now, but truly, how many times have you blown off a yoga class or coffee date with a friend to aimlessly browse the stores? We've already covered how shopping is not the emotional balm it advertises itself to be, and with a capsule wardrobe, you're going to Maxine Waters the hell out of this consumerist culture and reclaim your time. And if you're worried that a minimal wardrobe equals boring, please remember that French women, oft cited as the apex of style, rock significantly smaller closets than American gals. So we're all going to survive this in style, okay?

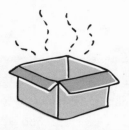

YOUR PAINLESS CLOSET DETOX

The springboard to closet nirvana is a good old-fashioned detox—a quick and dirty way to drill down to your priorities, minimize accordingly, and fight the man (because, let's face it, the only folks who win from our shopping addictions and habits are the exact people and organizations who don't give a shit about you or the environment—just their profits). And the good news is that it doesn't have to hurt—in fact, it feels really freaking awesome. A few small shifts in your approach to acquiring clothing and taking stock of your wardrobe needs will save your sanity, time, and wallet while also making a big impact on the planet.

Getting Started

There's nothing quite as liberating as clearing the cobwebs of emotional purchases—aspirational jeans, too-small shoes, forgotten shirts with tags still on 'em—and winnowing down to only the stuff you wear and love. But I get it: the thought of tackling that behemoth of a closet can be, well, terrifying. Don't fret! Though I'm not physically there with you, I've created this fun and foolproof guide to get you pared down and on your way in three hours flat. And if you're feeling overwhelmed or like you need me there, just head to the bathroom, hit the lights, and say my name three times in the mirror. (Kidding—I am not a witch, but I am working on it.)

What You'll Need

Prepare thyself:

→ Hangers (I like wood and metal ones because they're durable and sustainable, but if you already have a bunch of plastic ones, use what you've got)

→ Mobile app for making lists (I like Wunderlist)

→ One storage container or bin with lid (you probably have a few of these kicking around your house, so repurpose one or something else you already have)

→ Three large reusable bags

→ A full-length mirror

→ Vacuum or broom/dustpan and cleaner for closet and drawers

→ A kickass playlist

→ Three whole, unadulterated hours to yourself (no skimping on this)

STEP 1: MAP YOUR STYLE + DETERMINE YOUR NUMBER

Time: 45 minutes

The traditional capsule wardrobe is around thirty-some odd pieces. However, different lives call for different accoutrements, so select a digit that's right for you by mapping out how you spend your time and the attendant wardrobe demands.

For instance, my estimates are as follows:

→ 50 percent—work, where I can dress casually (*hallelujah!*)

→ 40 percent—social and sleep, where I can wear whatever I darn well please

→ 10 percent—special occasion, where I need to have a killer dress to bring all the boys to the yard or a special ensemble that looks good on camera

Once you map out your activities (don't forget sports/exercise, volunteering, hobbies . . .), allocate how many of each item you'll need based on the season. For instance, a summer capsule may include a few swimsuits, sandals, a cover-up, and a permagrin, while a winter capsule, depending on where you live, may feature scarves, boots, gloves, hats, and a resting bitch face that clearly communicates your disdain for frigid temps.

Remember your basics too. Unless you're gifted with a body that needs no underpinnings, you're going to need bras, underwear, socks, the occasional tights, and maybe even shapewear. Factor those in, and make your number robust enough to accommodate real-life needs without allowing too many emotional inclusions to creep in. For instance, my summer capsule looked like:

- One pair black cigarette pants
- Two pairs skinny jeans, 1 blue and 1 black (I don't do shorts)
- One pair boyfriend jeans (or whatever those too-big, ripped-up jeans are called)
- Two blazers
- One versatile day/work dress
- One formal dress
- One pencil skirt
- One pair heels
- One swimsuit
- One cover-up/kaftan
- One pair Swedish-type clog shoes that make me feel stylish but probably make my legs look like tree trunks
- One midweather jacket
- One jean jacket
- Three V-neck T-shirts
- Two concert T-shirts (The Smiths and Tears for Fears, if you're wondering)
- One pair running shoes
- Two pairs sandals
- One pair flats
- Three pairs yoga pants

- Three workout tops
- Two sports bras
- Five pairs socks
- Five bras
- One pair tights
- One pair shapewear (because i like to eat at weddings)
- One pair pajamas

- Eight versatile tops (button-downs and blouses that are appropriate for both work and kickin' around town)
- One clutch bag
- One work bag
- One cross-body bag
- One backpack

That's a total of fifty-seven articles of clothing. That's still a fuck ton in capsule wardrobe land, guys. Also, Ashlee, where's your underwear? Um, well, I don't wear any, so now you know even more about me than you ever wanted to know. Bye.

STEP 2: THE PURGE
Time: 1:30

My advice probably flies in the face of that of organization experts who suggest that people attack clutter little by little. But if you're anything like me, that will *not* work. I usually get rid of two shirts, only to incorporate four new ones in the mix. Party fail. Besides, this is a detox. You don't embark on a five-day juice cleanse with a side of hoagies, right? So I recommend taking everything out of the closet. Yep, *all of it*. If you have a ton of stuff (you know who you are), this may take you longer than the time allotted. And if that's the case, let us take a moment to bless up because that is an extremely fortunate problem to have. And why a time limit, you ask? Well, this should be an unemotional process. The longer you have to reminisce about how you thought you'd wear that dress that is two sizes too small to your high school reunion (points to self), the less likely you are to purge it. And we are here to go scorched earth on your closet. Before you purge your wardrobe, set out the storage bin and ready the reusable bags because they have a purpose:

→ The storage bin is for out-of-season items that you want to store.

→ Reusable bag 1 is for items you're keeping that need repairs.

→ Reusable bag 2 is for items you don't want that you will either consign or swap among pals (more on both of those topics later in the chapter, BTW).

→ Reusable bag 3 is for items you're donating.

As you remove items from the closet and drawers, create piles based upon type—pants, shoes, shirts, dresses, and so on. The consideration process should look like this:

→ If an item is out of season (i.e., winter coat, boots, sweater dress) but you still love or need it, put it in the storage bin you have ready, and hide it away until its season arrives.

→ Items you love but require a little TLC (like replacing buttons, darning small holes, or giving a good cleaning) go into bag 1.

→ If an item is too big, too small, or isn't your jam anymore but is of good quality to resell or pass to a friend, put it in bag 2 (items deemed too wonky for bag 2 automatically go to bag 3 for donation).

→ Any remaining items in the piles you should try on in front of a mirror (it helps to have a brutally honest friend or small child with no filter around). If something doesn't fit, looks weird, or doesn't make you feel like a million bucks, don't let it make its way back into the closet, and send it to the appropriate bag.

Remember, you don't need to meet all your capsule targets with your existing clothes. It's awesome if you can, but if you don't have the right item right now, you can always acquire it using my guidelines for ethical purchases, which I'll get to in a moment.

STEP 3:
SAVOR THE SPACE

Time: 45 minutes

This may be one of the few times you have a blissfully clear closet, so bust out the vacuum, clear away the dust bunnies, and clean that bad boy top to bottom. Then lovingly hang and fold the items that made the cut and neatly arrange them. Burn some sage, do a dance, get crazy, christen the space with wild lovemaking, take a shot. You've earned it.

Bag 1: Repairing

You needn't know how to operate a sewing machine or spend your weekends weaving fabric to keep your wardrobe in good repair. Because a big part of having a more conscious closet is taking good care of what you've got, you only need to embrace a few basics of wardrobe maintenance.

→ **Address and maintain**: Stains and tears get worse the longer you leave them unaddressed, so it's best to tackle them when they first happen. Moreover, regular upkeep will ensure your duds are always wear-worthy. Maintenance doesn't need to be arduous or require a billion expensive tools. Remove pills from sweaters and the inner thighs of pants with a dry razor or porous foot file. Condition and treat leathers with simple oils, balms, and a reusable cloth (hey, if you already have leather goods, I'm not judging and would certainly rather you make them last as long as possible). Deodorize and dry out sweaty shoes with cornstarch and a few drops of essential oil. Give dingy cloth sneakers new life with a hot-water soak. The options for vitalizing your garments and accessories are endless and don't require you to take out a loan or cancel your weekend plans.

→ **Get good people**: As is true with any aspect of life, delegating to reliable professionals to fill in the blanks where you're not adept is the key to success. In this case, we're talking tailors and cobblers. These long-revered professionals will blow your mind with their messiah-like abilities to make all things new again. Tailors are fabulous for altering secondhand clothing, hemming, fixing buttons and zippers, mending holes and lining, and even turning items you no longer need (bridesmaid's dress) into something you actually want (sexy LBD). Cobblers can resole shoes; fix heels, insoles, and straps; stretch too-small kicks to fit; and polish dingy materials. Many can even fix broken bag handles and stitching. These magicians will be your ticket to keeping your duds alive and kicking for years to come.

Bag 2: Consigning and Swapping

This bag should contain items that are clean and in good repair (and if they're not, get them there) but simply don't work for you anymore because of fit, size, style, bad memories—whatever the reason. Also, pay special attention to any designer brands you have lurking in your wardrobe because we're gonna be selling these bad boys, and the people go crazy for resale Chanel and the like. There's an art and an order to addressing the items in this bag, and it goes a little something like this: (1) Take all the hot-to-trot items therein to your fave consignment store (check out reviews and get recommendations from in-the-know friends if you're not sure where to start), and see what you can get for them (don't worry—I'll show you how in a sec). (2) If anything isn't purchased by the first store, you can opt to sell to another store (I have three near each other I hit up in sequential order on the regular), or hedge your bets selling online through eBay, Craigslist, ThredUp, or Poshmark. (3) Any items remaining after steps one and two? Bring 'em to your next clothing swap (more on that in a minute).

CONSIGNMENT

There are few (legal) ways to make money these days that don't involve a nine-to-five gig or donating an essential body fluid. Thankfully, selling your gently used clothes and accessories is an easy way to responsibly rid your closet of stuff you no longer love while putting some extra jingle in your pocket. I personally love my monthly sojourn to my local Crossroads Trading consignment place, where I bring a few items, they give me cash, and I turn right around and spend said cash on something secondhand and dope I find in the store. Symbiosis at its finest. And although consigning used to be a luxury limited to designer brands, now options for swapping any brand clothing for dolla-dolla bills are plentiful. Explore the storefront consignment and resale options in your area. Many will offer you a price on the spot for your items, while others will do a true consignment model, which gives you a percent payout once the item has sold. I suggest getting your items in their cleanest, best condition before going there and, in the case of my local store, maybe dress like you kind of have style, because I find they're way nicer to me and more likely to buy my shit if I don't wear my pajamas and smudged night-before eye makeup.

Moreover, online options for turning clothes to cash are everywhere. Although packing and shipping are usually required—making online a less eco-friendly option than in-store consigning—outlets from Poshmark and ThredUp to eBay and Craigslist make transforming your trash into someone's treasure so freaking easy. For more options, check out ashleepiper.com/LBB.

SWAP TILL YOU DROP

Forgive me if I sound like your neighbor who drones on about how he was the first person ever to use the internet, but I've legit been hosting clothing swaps for fifteen-plus years. Yes, that makes me sound old, but it also makes me sound awesome. The formula for a dope swap is shockingly simple: cool people (ideally around twenty attendees of all ages, shapes, sizes, and styles) + booze = legendary swap. That's it, really. Sometimes I mix in some light bites and good tunes, but no more. I always (1) get amazing new-to-me stuff and (2) meet awesome new friends-of-friends at a swap. In addition to being eco-friendly and a great opportunity to give a haul to charity, a well-done swap can be a real boon to anyone's social circle. I once left a swap with a vintage yellow bicycle, Ferragamo slippers, and a date with an attendee's totally smokin' brother who turned out to be a really great guy. True story. Forget Disney—miracles happen at the clothing swap, kids.

The term *swap* isn't really accurate because this isn't like the old school swap meets at the trading post where everyone had to bring something to get something. I tell peeps to bring whatever they're looking to off-load—clothes, accessories, beauty products (perhaps one of the only acceptable places to off-load sanitized used eye shadows and lipsticks), home goods, books, kitchen stuff, décor, whatever—and come with reusable bags so they can take what they want. Then, after everyone's arrived, set up their items in designated areas, gotten good and sauced, and taken whatever they want, I donate all that remains to appropriate charities. Sometimes, if you're sly like a fox, you can find consignment-worthy castoffs in the leftovers. But you didn't hear that from me.

SELLING YOUR SKIVVIES

Oh, look. It's another "do as I say, not as I do" tale of poor judgment. Fun. A while back (like a week ago) my friend Alisha and I were approaching a busy coffee shop, bags of shoes and clothes in tow. We were nervous. Why? Well, a few weeks prior she posted her wedding dress for sale on Craigslist. A dude offered a crazy amount of money to buy it and also posited that he would offer similar dough for other, more delicate lady clothes items.

Being the enterprising woman of the world that I am, I immediately offered up my ratty old unmentionables (that would otherwise end up in the landfill, so there's eco-motivation here, guys), and said dude rose to the occasion by offering a bananas sum for the haul. Now, although I admit it's a tad unorthodox to relinquish one's skivvies to a complete stranger and may come back to haunt me when I run for public office (but hell, this whole book will do that, so . . .), I felt this was both compassionate (people have fetishes—who am I to judge?), sustainable (I'm sparing the landfill), and businesswoman-like (because I was going to get $900 for four old bras and some pantyhose), and I just prayed the guy wasn't a voodoo priest who would make a doll of my underpinnings and fuck up my life forever.

We waited at that coffee shop for an hour, on high alert, and he never showed. What is the moral of this story, you ask? Well, don't sell your underwear to a stranger, maybe? Or at least bring a friend if you do? That botched attempt aside, the fortunate truth is that you can make big bucks selling your clothes, and you don't even have to broker deals with faceless, nameless men to get the cash. And if you want to buy my bras, hit me up on Instagram.

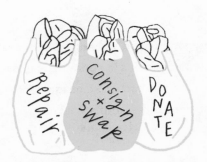

Bag 3: Donating

I used to hate litterbugs with a passion. I mean, I still do, but the new wave of litterbugs isn't the defiant kids tossing soda bottles into the street—it's the people who throw clothes and other items that can easily be donated in the dang trash. In addition to being a thoughtless way of dealing with unwanted items, I consider this gratuitous trashing to be an indication of a gross lack of imagination. (*Hmm, who could possibly use this winter coat I no longer wear? In a midwestern January?*) The truth is that there's literally a legit and very rad donation outlet for pretty much anything. The creepy fur coat collection bequeathed to you by Aunt Lidia? Well, it can be donated to certain wildlife sanctuaries to help orphaned animals feel like they're cuddled up to Mama (just call ahead to ensure they're still open to such donations). Those sneakers that saw you through the marathon? Give them to programs that empower persons experiencing homelessness through running, like Back on My Feet. Oh, and those transition-lens specs that rather unfortunately made you look like a pedophile? Optometrists will fix 'em up and distribute them to the visually impaired in developing countries. Even used underwear and socks can have a little extra life prelandfill by being ripped into strips, tied to a rope, and made into a chew toy for your dog (he's gonna go for them anyway). Be thoughtful about how you can offload, opting for reuse and resale before donating, and if you need ideas, boy howdy, I have an entire page on my website that shows you how and where you can ethically repurpose and offload pretty much anything (check it, ashleepiper.com/ethicaloffload).

BUILDING YOUR KIND CLOSET

So by now you might have actually cleaned your closet and responsibly rehomed the items you no longer need. If you haven't gotten there yet, that's okay—you're still allowed to read on (you're welcome). This section is of the use-any-time-you-dang-well-please ilk. So although it's best when paired with a squeaky-clean closet, as directed above, I'm about to arm you with knowledge you can rock anytime you set out to acquire clothes or accessories. Sound good? Good.

FOLLOW THE THREADS

If you were told as a youngster that it's impolite to ask people pressing questions, I'm going to give you permission right now to banish that stinkin' thinkin'. A big part of giving a shit is inquiring and thinking critically beyond the information readily provided. Whether you're researching your next shoe splurge or a new lipstick shade, if you're not quite sure about the ethical ethos of the company or transparency in manufacturing, by golly, ASK. What does that look like? Well, sometimes it looks like scouring a company's FAQs and even calling the customer support line (plaid detective's cap optional). This may sound a little extra to some, but doing your due diligence gives you peace of mind and also shows companies that the virtues about which you're inquiring are important. This is largely how cruelty-free cosmetics and conscious collections at major retailers got their start: people became less lazy and more inquisitive. And when they received answers they didn't like ("yep, we test on animals") or that seemed too cryptic to be conclusive ("to our knowledge, we do not employ child labor . . ."), they stopped buying from that company. Imagine how quickly companies and the world would change if we took a hot second to do that! Consumers are the lifeblood of fashion companies, so never underestimate the important role your feedback plays in turning the tide.

Secondhand First

I know I'm starting to sound like a broken record, but really, secondhand clothing and accessories are the gentlest options on the planet for the simple reason that they already exist. Can you find the item you're yearning for at a consignment, resale, or thrift store? And we all know those effortlessly stylish people who, when asked where they got that insanely rad necklace or blazer, nonchalantly respond, "Oh this? It's vintage." Shopping secondhand first means that *you can be that person*. Plus, the likelihood of you rolling up to a party wearing the same outfit as your frenemy is very slim when you shop from the timeless and abundant universe of resale.

The Ethical Edit

As is the case with toothbrushes and underwear, sometimes new is just the most socially acceptable way to go. And that's cool, especially because the following definitions mean you won't be buying blind. So, as with anything in this book, arm yourself with the knowledge, prioritize what virtues are important to and possible for you, and go to town creating an ethically edited wardrobe you can be proud of. Treat welcoming new items into your closet a bit like the search for true love: when you've found something that makes you go all emoji-with-heart-eyes for its look, feel, and, most importantly, embodiment of wonderful, sound values, you know it'll be an everlasting love.

Language around fair labor can be tricky, so due diligence is required to see which companies are using the nimble fingers of children to sew their threads and which give a flying shit about people's well-being. That said, the following terms and certifications can be good North Stars in ensuring you're supporting business practices aligned with your social justice values:

Fair trade: Duds meet standards that ensure ethical practices from sourcing to manufacturing to shipping set forth by the Fair Trade Certified seal. Workers at all levels are at will (not forced), paid fairly, and work in safe and regulated conditions.

Community development: This term means an item supports or is a product of micro-loan programs, cooperatives, employee- and female-ownership models, and rehabilitation and retraining programs (think: reentering incarcerated peeps or women escaping sexual slavery). These programs not only give workers an empowering socioeconomic stake in their craft but also support the development of stronger, safer communities where the items are produced.

Charitable: Whether it's an in-kind, get-one-give-one model (like Tom's shoes); a proceeds percentage donation; or a commitment to plant trees for every item sold, companies with these models in place make a point to give back. Supporting companies with these beliefs and practices is a great way to give a shit while doing things you already do.

SUSTAINABLE MATERIALS

Natural fibers and innovations in high-tech materials (think faux suede and durable, downy insulation made from recycling plastic bottles, for instance) will blow your mind whilst helping our spinning ecosystem. Consider these material options the gold standard in your fabric selections:

Natural: Limit resource-guzzling synthetics like polyester, nylon, and acrylic, and opt for organic and more readily biodegradable materials like untreated, pesticide-free cotton; linen; hemp; jute; bamboo; and raffia. Natural materials break down more gently and introduce fewer foreign chemicals into our soil and waterways. This is important because a recent sample of global tap water found that 83 percent contained harmful microplastic fibers, and that ain't cute.[16]

Semisynthetic: If you must go synthetic, options like rayon/viscose, modal, and Lyocell/Tencel are gentler options.

Reclaimed and recycled: You can't beat utilizing materials already in existence, so garments boasting words like repurposed, recycled, refashioned, reclaimed, upcycled, and a percentage of postconsumer waste mean that some form of the holy "reduce, reuse, recycle" adage has been woven into production.

Nontoxic: Opt for items made with natural vegetable or azo-free dyes and adhesives.

Organic: Materials are mostly or completely free from nonnatural pesticides, insecticides, herbicides, and fertilizers that can harm ecosystems and workers.

GREEN PRACTICES

How a garment is produced is just as important as the materials from which it's made. The following practices are gentler on the environment, and some even give you options to recycle or replace your used clothing so they don't make their way to a trashy grave.

Zero waste: An estimated 15 percent of global textile waste comes from scraps generated by garment manufacturing.[17] Traditional factories work at breakneck speed with large swathes of material and wasteful patterns, thereby tossing loads of scraps before products even reach the consumer. Zero-waste fashion utilizes efficient patterns and salvaged or upcycled materials to create little to no waste at the pre- and postconsumer levels.

Renewable energy: Look for companies that power production with alternative energy like wind and solar as well as transport goods via electric or hybrid means. Many companies also offset their resource utilization by planting trees, purchasing carbon-offset credits, or by supporting sustainable community development efforts.

Buy-back and recycling programs: In addition to offering repairs to extend the life of garments, companies like Patagonia and Eileen Fisher also have postconsumer disposal or buy-back programs that will either resell or recycle your used items.

ANIMAL FRIENDLY

Even if you're not ready to give up bacon, you can still make a big impact on the planet and our animal pals by curating a cruelty-free closet.

TRANSCEND THE TAG

Some items simply don't have materials labels. And because few among us are animal fur or skin experts, ensuring that purchases without symbols are critter-free can be a mystery. The following manufacturing symbols can help you determine whether those faux leather shoes, for instance, have deal-breaker suede heel cups or soles.

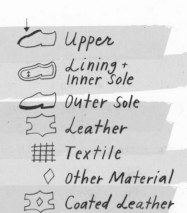

Upper

Lining + Inner Sole

Outer Sole

Leather

Textile

Other Material

Coated Leather

Vegan: A term that used to garner eye rolls and spite in the fashion industry, vegan fashion has now become a popular choice for even high-end brands (not to mention legitimately fashionable). Look for symbols and awards like "PETA-Approved" and "Vegan" for assurance that items were not produced with any animal materials or byproducts (sneakier ones like glues and adhesives made from boiled-down animal connective tissues, though rare, can be a real bummer). Moreover, companies like Toms, Patagonia, Asos, Free People, and Urban Outfitters have online sections dedicated to vegan wares. And if you're worried that animal-friendly boots or bags are going to make you look like a fashion reject, I have two words for you: Stella McCartney.

Faux: Be careful with this one, kiddos. A 2014 Humane Society of the United States undercover investigation found that Chinese-produced, major-label garments sold at US retailers claiming to have "faux" fur trim were actually found to be made with DOG FUR, a common regulatory dupe, especially in countries like China, where human and animal rights standards are poor.[18]

LOCAL

Considering how far finished garments and materials travel is an important part of making the eco-friendliest acquisitions. Given the distance between where most fast fashion is produced (developing countries) and sold (Western countries), a lot of ships, trains, planes, and attendant fuel and pollution are required to get those items in store or to your door. Shopping locally, even in the form of Made in the USA items, can support smaller makers better able to control (and explain to you) their materials, suppliers, and manufacturing processes. It also means your beloved garment didn't do more world traveling than a college senior finding himself whilst backpacking through Europe.

QUICK HITS
IN YOUR CLOSET

Sure, the fastest way to ace ethical wardrobing might seem like joining a nudist colony, but until you (and everyone around you) are ready for that, these five-minute fixes will keep you consciously clothed.

- *Examine your closet and see what you actually wear. Commit to simply turning the hangers around on the items you've worn over the course of a month, and reevaluate thereafter.*

- *Research secondhand and consignment stores in your area. Ask friends and your social media fam which are their favorites. And if you've never been, plan a trip to peruse.*

- *Look at your bank account. How many clothing items have you purchased over the past ninety days that were necessity versus impulse? Then add up how much you spent on the impulse purchases. If the number has you sweating bullets, perhaps it's time to consider the Give a Shit Closet Detox.*

- *Pick a date and plan a clothing swap (guidance on page 194). Prepare for mega fun.*

- *If you've got a hot date or a fancy function, ask around your networks to see if you can borrow a more special occasion outfit as opposed to buying something new. It'll be like a ritzy version of the Sisterhood of the Traveling Pants.*

- *The next time you pass a fast-fashion retailer, eye the display windows, but don't go in. Resisting mindless consumption is a muscle that gets stronger the more it's tested and exercised. If you're a chronic shopper, consider this the dumbbells portion of the mental workout.*

Give a Shit:

In the Mirror

We live in some interesting times. On the daily we are inundated with advertising that pushes us to believe that to attain a weirdly prescribed standard of beauty (and that if you're not lithe with perfect skin, hair, and lips that are pouty even sans makeup, well, you're not trying hard enough). This daily assault isn't new and has been compounded to near-epidemic, can't-escape-it-giving-you-hives levels with the surge in social media. Seriously. Unless you're living in a cave, you're bombarded with thousands of sales pitches and beauty dictates every day. No matter how strong and impervious you may be, this can start to affect your purchasing choices. (Ever rack up a $150 tab at Sephora without even thinking? Yeah. That.) Moreover, these messages aren't just selling us an impossible standard of beauty; they're also selling us the attendant seedy, very fugly processes that go into creating the products that are supposed to make us beautiful. From unpronounceable toxic chemicals that can cause illness, to animal testing that unnecessarily harms sweet critters, to wasteful packaging and nonbiodegradable formulas that pollute our planet indefinitely, the beauty and personal care industries behave as if they have an all-access pass to our wallets and our self-esteem, and most of the time they're happy to exploit this monopoly with little remorse.

Hold your head up high, though! All is not doomed. When armed with the right information, you can make much healthier decisions for your own beauty and environmental standards. And I'm already confident that you're a hip cat because you picked up this book, so obviously you have rad taste and care and all that good stuff. To that end, this chapter will assist you in demystifying (and perhaps even joyfully embracing) the following topics so you can be your own beauty boss, pesky corporate marketing be damned:

> **The anatomy of the label**: How to decipher symbology and attendant meanings as well as what to look for and what to avoid when you're in the beauty aisle. This includes how to shop with confidence for vegan, cruelty-free, and organic products.

> **Paring down to make up**: An easy checklist that will help everyone—from the most die-hard beauty junkie to the cosmetics averse—create a minimalist routine that works in simple, eco-friendly steps.

> **When in doubt, BYOB (build your own beauty)**: A series of my favorite, tried-and-true DIY recipes that will save you money and the planet—and, of course, keep you radiant and smelling like someone people wanna get close to.

Now, don't freak out. I'm not going to suggest you throw out your eighty-seven lip glosses and cede your Sephora VIB platinum card to become a bare-faced, coconut-oil-for-everything kind of person (unless that's what you want). Nah. As with all the advice in this book, I aim to give you the information and tips so you can pick and choose what works for you as you build your own personal blueprint for being the most gorgeously green version of you. Besides, as a semireformed product junkie (a friend once said my primary food group was lipstick), I believe that you can have both—the delight of high-performance products that enhance, transform, and pamper as well as the relief that comes from a more minimalist, natural, compassionate routine.

ANIMAL TESTING (IS BULLSHIT)

This is one area where you won't hear me take the laissez faire "you do you, pal" approach. Why? Well, my personal philosophy has always revolved around this basic guideline: Hurt yourself? That's silly (but ultimately your prerogative). Hurt someone else? You're a dick. Animal testing, also known as vivisection, falls very squarely into the latter category.

You're probably shocked that animal testing for cosmetics purposes still happens in the United States. Like, did we time travel back one hundred years to when doctors were committing people to institutions for masturbating? Nope. Unlike in countries like China, animal testing for cosmetics and household products isn't actually required by the FDA or the US Consumer Products Safety Commission. In fact, these organizations support the development and use of humane alternatives. Why the heck, then, do more than an estimated one hundred million guinea pigs, rabbits, mice, rats, and other sweet, sweet creatures needlessly suffer and die in labs each year for our home cleaners and shampoos?[1] Welp, some

LAB LIFE SUCKS

If you're thinking vivisection is just lathering up some rabbits with bubble bath, allow me to shed some light on what animal testing is actually like. According to the Humane Society of the United States, routine tests for cosmetics and home products include:

* *Rubbing chemicals into animals' eyes and skin to measure and determine irritation*

* *Force-feeding substances to animals to establish whether said ingredients cause cancer and other illnesses*

* *Controversial but still in existence "lethal dose" tests that involve forced dosing with the express purpose of causing death*

Oh, and animals are usually restrained, fucking terrified (duh), and given no painkillers. Lab life is lonely and stressful; the tests bring about suffering, sickness, and are often fatal; and, in some cases, undercover footage has captured lab workers abusing, starving, and neglecting animal subjects. At the end of a testing trial, many animals are killed without pain relief, usually by neck breaking, asphyxiation, or decapitation. Modern-day animal testing (which kinda sounds like medieval torture, huh?) is some fucked-up shit.

companies develop new ingredients and think that animal tests are bioidentical enough to prove their efficacy and safety. I don't know about you, but last time I checked, I'm not a rat, and those little guys are gorgeous all on their own without lipstick. Moreover, breeding animals for testing labs is an entrenched industry unto itself, and many companies are just too dang lazy or don't feel consumer pressure (and attendant profit loss) to explore humane alternatives. Let that latter statement put the fire in your belly to write, call, tweet, and fucking send Morse code messages companies your insistence that they jump on those nonanimal alternatives ASAP.

Real talk: animal testing has little to no merit in modern-day cosmetics. More scientifically sterling humane options exist that don't use animals at all. Computer simulators and testing on artificial, lab-grown human tissue have yielded more accurate results on predicting skin irritation than animal tests.[2] Vivisection for cosmetics has already been banned in more than thirty-eight major economies, like Israel, India, and the European Union.[3] Although the United States is woefully behind on doing the right thing, thankfully the market is flooded with totally awesome cruelty-free products that give you all the looks, performance, and fun of traditional animal-tested versions.

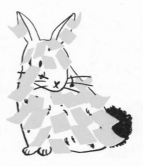

WHAT IN THE ACTUAL FUCK?

Now that we've firmly established that animal testing is bananas, get ready to have your mind blown by these everyday items that can be tested on critters. I have a pretty vivid imagination, and even I can't fathom why (or how) these items are tested on innocent animals:

- ✳ *Post-it Notes*
- ✳ *bandages*
- ✳ *garbage bags*
- ✳ *batteries*
- ✳ *condoms*
- ✳ *diapers*
- ✳ *contact lenses*
- ✳ *razors*
- ✳ *furniture polish*

Lemme turn that frown upside down for a minute. A quick website scan, call, or email to your favorite company can usually get you the answers you need to buy with confidence. And if their responses are nonexistent or feel sketchy, I've included awesome companies at ashleepiper.com/LBB to give you all the intel you need to purchase with cruelty-free confidence.[ii]

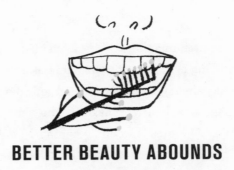

BETTER BEAUTY ABOUNDS

Seriously, cruelty-free options are like fanny packs at Disneyland—EVERYWHERE. Check it out: I was recently road tripping from Chicago to Dallas with my pup. The journey is long but gives me lots of good thinking and singing-songs-loudly-without-other-people-scowling-at-me time. One particular two-hour stretch of this sojourn goes through mostly small towns in rural Oklahoma. After ten consecutive hours on the road, I was getting pretty tired, so I pulled over at a run-of-the-mill truck stop to fill my reusable mug with hot coffee and to freshen up. As I opened my bag, I realized I'd left my toothpaste at home. But I was pleasantly surprised to peruse the dust-crusted aisles and find Tom's of Maine toothpaste staring me in the face, comforting Leaping Bunny symbol and all.

Moral of the story? If I can find a kinder toothpaste in the middle of nowhere in a pinch, we can all sure as hell source cruelty-free products no matter where we live, whether it's at an ethical chain, a local business, or ye olde worldwide web and make that shit happen. And if you're afraid of the internet, I've included some recipes for my favorite personal care staples that don't involve you brushing your teeth with a stick.

Basically, no excuses. Each time you think of one (and usually they're really silly), imagine yourself saying it to a terrified, restrained rabbit being force-fed some toxic ingredient du jour, and check yourself before you wreck loads of animals' lives.

SHANGHAI, AND BYE

Perhaps the most buzzed-about happening in the realm of vivisection was the decision of some formerly cruelty-free companies to sell in China. Why is this buzz worthy? Well, China mandates animal testing for certain products sold in the country, even if the company is strictly cruelty-free. This means that in order to expand into the nearly $30 billion Chinese cosmetics market, companies have to concede to the Chinese government conducting animal tests on their products. It is estimated that each year more than 375,000 animals die in China for cosmetics testing alone. While advancements in nonanimal testing methodologies and public pressure signal a lessened reliance on animal testing in China and worldwide, props to good guys like Paul Mitchell and LUSH, who stay true to their cruelty-free stance by hard passing on the opportunity to sell in China.[iii]

Spotting the Good Guys

After all that sadness, you're probably chomping at the bit to find out how you can avoid supporting this madness at all costs. And you're in luck, because sourcing critter-friendly products is easy if you know what to look for. But because protecting animals also means avoiding ingredients procured by animal exploitation, this symbology grid also includes vegan designations so your regimen can be free from the creepy shit that typically makes its way into products. Ingredients like allantoin (a moisturizer sourced from cow urine), carmine (red coloring made from crushed beetle shells), collagen and elastin (skin cream additives derived from animal bones, connective tissues, and placentas), tallow (animal fat commonly used in soap), and squalene (shark liver oil) are widely used and, as you can gather, are either by-products of animal suffering like agricultural slaughter or directly cause animal trauma and death.[4] Plus, urine on your face? No thanks.

Here's a helpful chart describing symbols and certifications you might see on beauty and personal care products and what it all means.

SYMBOL	PROGRAM	WHAT IT MEANS
Leaping Bunny logo	Leaping Bunny	Companies and ingredient suppliers do not conduct or commission animal tests.
Cruelty free bunny symbol	PETA Beauty without Bunnies	Companies and their ingredient suppliers do not conduct, commission, or pay for any animal tests for ingredients, formulations, or finished products.
Not Tested on Animals Rabbit logo	Choose Cruelty Free (Australia)	In at least five years prior to certification, products and ingredients are not tested on animals by the company, nor have suppliers or third parties conducted tests on the company's behalf. Some restrictions on animal ingredients.
Certified Vegan logo	Vegan Action	Products contain no animal ingredients, by-products, or animal testing conducted or commissioned at any point, by any party, during sourcing or formulation.
Vegan sunflower logo	Vegan Society	Products contain no animal ingredients, by-products, or animal testing conducted or commissioned at any point, by any party, during sourcing or formulation.

Some rules of thumb when shopping for animal-friendly stuff:

→ **Cruelty-free ≠ vegan and vice versa**: Cruelty-free and vegan are not mutually exclusive practices or terms. Products can bear a cruelty-free designation and still contain animal ingredients, and vegan goods can still be tested on animals. If you're passionate about supporting truly animal-friendly products, it's best to read labels (many animal ingredients have a host of scientific ingredient names employed interchangeably, so look them up or contact the company to be sure), and opt for goodies that have both vegan and cruelty-free designations.

→ **Actions (and symbols) speak louder than words**: Beware products bearing cryptic language and zero certifications. You see, in order to earn the certs above, companies usually need to have transparent sourcing and formulation, endure routine audits, and spend money. It's a lot of work, and when a company is legitimately cruelty-free or vegan, by golly, they—and their packaging—are gonna shout it from the freaking rooftops. If you find yourself holding a product—especially from a company known for vivisection—bearing lingo like "natural," "this finished product not tested on animals," "cruelty free," "suitable for vegetarians," and other BS-sounding phrases with none of the above accompanying symbols, think twice. Sure, there are some smaller, well-meaning businesses that have yet to get or afford the certifications, which they'll happily tell you if you contact them and ask. Or in the case of everyone's favorite bath bomb purveyor, LUSH, their products do not bear a traditional cruelty-free symbol from the facing chart because the company has its own standards for cruelty-free sourcing, formulation, monitoring, and even activism that are arguably more stringent than traditional designations. And they, like other well-meaning companies, will be delighted to tell you all about it if only you inquire.[5] But because phrases around animal treatment are largely unregulated (aside from the stamps of approval on the facing chart), marketers can claim whatever they think will inspire the false confidence required to make a sale. So call the companies, do your homework, and crowdsource the information before you buy.[6]

→ **Go beyond beauty**: These certifications are used in more than just cosmetics, so look for these symbols when you purchase feminine products and sexual protection, homeopathic remedies, home cleaners and supplies, baby care, and even clothes and accessories.

OTHER SHIT TO LOOK FOR

Because cruelty-free and vegan are just two pillars of giving a shit in the mirror, you may want to keep your eyes out for these other elements (like limited or reusable packaging) and certs that give a product even more eco–street cred.

SYMBOL	PROGRAM	WHAT IT MEANS
USDA Organic	USDA	Product contains 95 percent certified organic agricultural ingredients, but do your homework to ensure the product has the most organic content possible.
EcoCert	European Certification Agency	The European certification echoing the USDA Organic standards
Soil Association COSMOS Natural	Soil Association	European standard for products that are of mostly natural origin, but are not organic, are produced with no animal testing, genetically modified ingredients, EU-deemed controversial chemicals, parabens and phthalates, or synthetic colors, dyes, or fragrances.
Soil Association COSMOS Organic	Soil Association	European standard for products that are of mostly organic origin, are produced with no animal testing, genetically modified ingredients, EU-deemed controversial chemicals, parabens and phthalates, or synthetic colors, dyes, or fragrances.
NSF Contains Organic Ingredients seal	NSF International	Products contain a minimum of 70 percent organic ingredients and adhere to labeling, formulation, and marketing requirements for "contains organic ingredients" claims. NSF/ANSI 305 requires that USDA National Organic Program (NOP) or EU equivalent certified ingredients be used.
Fair Trade Certified seal	Fair Trade	Certified ingredients, such as shea butter and coconut oil, are sourced through trading relationships rooted in good working conditions, open dialogue, transparency, and sustainability for those in the developing world.
"OTCO" or "Oregon Tilth" symbol	Oregon Tilth	Respected USDA Organic and NSF certifying organization

7, 8, 9

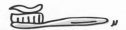

FAMILY MATTERS

Let's talk about parents for a sec—parent companies, that is. Many "green" companies are subsidiaries of larger companies that conduct animal tests. Tom's of Maine is owned by Colgate-Palmolive. Burt's Bees is owned by Clorox.[iv] Companies owning other companies is a normal occurrence in our capitalist world, and an offender parent company doesn't always mean the smaller brand is tested on animals, but if you're deeply concerned about what activities your money supports, it behooves you to get the skinny on who owns whom and if a company's cruelty-free stance will be maintained after the acquisition. This investigation is important because it also enables you to sidestep being "green washed," or duped into thinking that a product, due to imagery, advertising, or cryptic claims, is actually good for you, animals, and the planet. I literally LOL when I see ginormous animal testers releasing product lines boasting "green" and "natural" in the names. Don't be hoodwinked—many of these companies are simply pandering to consumer demand to keep your business without actually making systemic changes.

OTHER SHIT TO AVOID

Microbeads: These solid, round, small (less than 5mm in size) plastic particles are commonly used in cosmetics like scrubs and toothpastes. They're also huge culprits for global microplastic contamination. Every year in the United States an estimated eight trillion microbeads make their way to waterways, settle on the bottom of lakes and oceans, and are ingested by various organisms that mistake them for food.[10] These nondegradable polymers take freaking hundreds of years to break down. Although a US ban initiated by the Obama administration passed in 2016, a gradual phase-out (production halts by July 2017, sales of items containing micro-beads stop by July 2018, and, finally, over-the-counter sales of drugs containing microbeads end in July 2019) means that products containing these bastards will still be on shelves and in bathroom cabinets for a while.

Antibacterial anything: Americans have a borderline fanatical obsession with antibacterial everything, rooted largely in misinformation. I get it—other people can be totally gross. I ride the train every day, and although I love the idea of whirring through the city and enjoying architecture and the general urban din, I do not like having to watch people clip their nails or suck Dorito powder from their fingers on said train. It's enough to make you want to wear a silicone bodysuit and live in a hermetically sealed chamber. And marketers and manufacturers of antibacterial agents play upon our fears of contracting illnesses and taking in peoples' general grodiness by telling us, "Hey, cover yourself with this stuff because it kills all those germs." There are a few reasons this marketing ploy is bollocks. For one, all bacteria are not bad bacteria. Heck, some of those bugs are essential for keeping us healthy, and most of what we encounter every day doesn't bug us (see what I did there?) or have the potential to make us sick.[11]

Antibacterial soap isn't even that effective at accomplishing its intended purpose. In a 2016 ruling calling into question nineteen antibacterial agents, the FDA claimed there was insufficient evidence to prove that soaps and washes with antibacterial ingredients, such as triclosan and triclocarban, were "more effective than plain soap and water in preventing illness."[12] Hi, that's the FDA saying that, not your conspiracy theorist neighbor. Moreover, when bacteria are routinely exposed to antibacterial agents,

CLEAR THE AIR

From our laundry detergents to our cars, it's rare that we enter a space without being assaulted by some heavily perfumed cocktail of chemical scents. Now, I'm not against smelling good. Quite to the contrary. But if we're going to be eco-friendly, we need to get real about chemical air fresheners. First, there's a big difference between "smells kinda nice" and truly "aromatherapeutic." Chemical air fresheners can contain thousands of potentially carcinogenic ingredients.[v] One study of pregnant women showed a link between the use of air fresheners and an increase in head-aches and depression in the mothers as well as ear infections and diarrhea in their babies.[vi] Moreover, many air fresheners are tested on animals (which, yes, I know seems unfathomably ridiculous), pollute the environ-ment, and often feature excessive packaging that cannot be reused or properly recycled. So skip the sprays and plug-ins, and opt for options like:

❋ My badass homemade air (and stuff) freshener made by simply mixing water with your choice of essential oils. My fave: mix fifteen drops each of rosemary and lavender essential oils, seven drops of lemon essential oil, and one to one and a half cups of water together in a repurposed small glass or metal spray bottle. Simply shake before each spritz, and prepare for crazy clean-smelling air, clothes, people—everything.

❋ Natural, compostable incense sticks or cones. You can sometimes find these completely package-free at some health food stores.

❋ Dried herb bundles (like sage, rosemary, lavender, and thyme) and woods like palo santo. These don't burn as long as incense, but their earthy scents linger, and their ash is completely compostable and biodegradable.

❋ Soy candles. Just ensure that these beauties are naturally scented in minimal containers (or none, in the case of votive and pillar candles) that you can reuse.

❋ Essential oils. In a diffuser or scattered around like confetti. Whatever brings you olfactory joy, bro.

❋ Plants (you can read my ode to these air cleaners in the home section, page 50).

❋ A trusty box of matches. Light one, let it burn for a moment, and blow it out. Voilà, funky smell gone.

they can undergo genetic mutations. These mutations can make them immune to the antibacterial product you are using, making bacteria more difficult to kill with antibiotics (these super-annoying, mutated bacteria are also known as "superbugs"). Every time you lather up, antibacterial agents creep into waterways because most wastewater treatment facility processes cannot fully eliminate them.[13] Traces of triclosan, for instance, have been found in breastmilk and urine of 75 percent of Americans over the age of five.[14] Because many antibacterial agents become carcinogenic as they degrade, they've been linked to disrupted hormones, impaired muscle function, increased allergies, and weakened immune systems.[15] Do yourself a favor and switch to something simpler. I personally love the ease of getting lavender castile soap from my local bulk store. It works well for so many things (hand and body soap, dishwashing liquid, laundry detergent), has ingredients I can pronounce that assimilate safely into waterways, isn't tested on animals, and smells great without stripping the skin. That's, like, a five-way win, which no, is not the latest sexual craze.

PARE DOWN TO MAKE UP

Prepare for déjà vu because just as we minimized your home and wardrobe, part of giving a shit is also streamlining your grooming regimen so you use what you've got, buy less frivolously, and restock with values. I first challenged myself to a simplified routine a decade ago during a period of multifaceted transition. I'd just exited a long-term relationship, left a ho-hum job, and had two of my closest pals move to different cities across the country to put down roots and start families—all at the same time. To cope, I'd browse and buy makeup at an astonishing rate. Eventually I realized that I could use my newly reclaimed time to recalibrate who I wanted to be and what I needed to improve. This included acknowledging my product addiction and getting it under control with a beauty fast (the exact fast I present below, in fact). The results were life changing: my skin improved thanks to a simplified and consistent routine, people could pinpoint my "signature perfume" because I stuck with it, I spent less time getting ready, and I enjoyed (and actually finished) the products I had. I still employ this system today to keep my grooming routine blissfully simple and enjoyable.

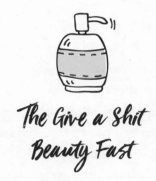

The Give a Shit Beauty Fast

Consider me your beauty bag sheriff. I may not have an old-timey moustache or smooth drawl, but I promise this approach will preserve sanity, save money, and lessen environmental burden without sacrificing your already head-turning good looks.

→ **Thirty for thirty**: Take stock of your desert-island grooming products—those items that really work and that you turn to repeatedly. Keep thirty items only. Put any extra stuff in a storage box or bag somewhere out of sight for a month. I recommend setting a calendar reminder on your phone to retrieve the box, because mark my words, you are going to forget about that shit. If in a month you find yourself desperately missing any of the stored items, I'll eat my hat. Here's my current not-so-dirty thirty (all this stuff is vegan and cruelty-free, FYI):

1. Shampoo bar in a reusable tin
2. Conditioner in a refillable bottle
3. Lavender castile soap
4. Turkish-style exfoliating mitt
5. Volumizing spray
6. Natural deodorant
7. Jojoba oil (for facial cleansing and moisturizing)
8. Reusable (and washable) cotton rounds
9. Hand/body lotion in a refillable metal bottle
10. Powdered toothpaste (not as freaky as it sounds)
11. Mostly compostable bamboo toothbrush
12. Lavender essential oil
13. Tea tree essential oil
14. Homemade dry shampoo
15. FSC-certified wood brush and a super-old plastic comb I've had since I was, like, twelve
16. Compostable cotton ear swabs
17. Safety razor with stainless-steel blade refills
18. Hair dryer
19. Curling iron
20. Metal and wood round brush
21. Nail care kit
22. Stainless-steel tweezers
23. Foundation in a recyclable tube
24. Concealer in a refillable compact
25. Mascara in a mostly recyclable tube

26. Black/brown eye pencil

27. Refillable neutral powder palette (that I use as contour and eye shadow)

28. Two lipsticks that double as blush (red and neutral pink) in recyclable containers

29. Homemade lip balm in a reusable jar

30. Perfume in a reusable glass bottle

→ **Clean up your act**: Few things feel as liberating as a tidy, organized space. So give your makeup bag or Dopp kit, tools, bathroom cabinet, products, and vanity a good once-over. Marvel at how light you feel when your morning doesn't consist of wrestling with a cabinet that won't shut or sifting through an overflowing bag of products.

→ **Abstain from buying replacements until your stuff is finished**: Yes, even the animal-tested crap you bought before you wised up. Relegating those items to the dumpster unused won't help the animals who suffered to bring it to market and will place extra burden on the environment. Also, when was the last time you finished a lipstick? My answer, after twenty years of wearing the stuff: never. Believe and trust that you will save money, time, and sanity by only replacing products when the ones you have in hand are completely donezo.

→ **Ethically restock**: Okay, you've used what you've got, so now the real fun begins. You know that "this is going to change my life" feeling certain beauty products inspire? Get ready to feel it again as you study up, sniff, sample, and enjoy the thrill of the hunt for products that align with your Give a Shit values.

→ **Or DIY**: You don't need to drop a mint on store-bought solutions to look and feel damn good. Sometimes making your own isn't just less expensive; it's more fun and functional. I've included easy recipes herein so you can dabble with creating effective eco-friendly products for pennies on the dollar.

Revamp Your Regimen

There's a Triple S (Simple Sustainable Swap) for almost every standard grooming item. Here are just a few of my faves to get you started:

TRADITIONAL TRASH MAKERS	SIMPLE SUSTAINABLE SWAPS
air fresheners	homemade versions; natural incense, herbs, and woods; essential oils; box of matches
antibacterial soap	liquid or bar castile soap
antifungal creams	tea tree oil
baby and body powder	cornstarch or arrowroot powder
body wash	liquid or bar castile soap
breath freshener	essential oils of spearmint, peppermint, or cinnamon (a few drops in the mouth get ya wicked fresh); sustainably harvested tea tree or cinnamon toothpicks
bubble bath and soaks	castile soap; Epsom and Dead Sea salts; essential oils; Soak Away the Sickies Bath soak (page 227)
conditioner	conditioner bars; cruelty-free and vegan options; natural oils and butters like coconut, avocado, and jojoba
contacts and contact solution	cruelty-free, minimally or recyclable-packaged contact solution; longest-wear contacts possible; or glasses because contacts are not recyclable
cosmetics	refillable options; cruelty-free, vegan options in recyclable or compostable packaging; permanent and semipermanent procedures and services (cruelty-free lash extensions, microblading, dyeing, tattooing); homemade versions
cotton balls, pads, and rounds	reusable, washable cotton rounds; compostable cotton balls

cotton swabs	metal ear cleaner; compostable cotton swabs
deodorant and antiperspirant	natural, cruelty-free, and vegan deodorants (skip antiperspirant—your body needs to sweat); homemade versions; baking soda; cornstarch; essential oils
dental floss	Waterpik; sustainably harvested toothpicks; unboxed floss not made from nylon
disposable feminine care	reusable options like menstrual cups, cloth pads, and period underwear
disposable nail file	reusable metal or glass versions
disposable razor or cartridges	reusable safety razor with refillable, recyclable blades; electric razor; waxing; electrolysis
dry shampoo	cornstarch or, better yet, my fab Declaration of Independence Dry Shampoo (page 226)
eyedrops	cruelty-free, minimally packaged versions
exfoliators	natural, nonmicrobead versions; homemade versions; reusable exfoliating mitt (my personal fave); terra-cotta or metal foot files
face wash	castile soap; micellar water; oil cleansers (try my Dewy Makeup-Removing Cleanser on page 225)
facial tissues	reusable, washable handkerchief
hair color	natural henna; cruelty-free and vegan versions; services at green, cruelty-free salons
hair growth treatments	castor oil (safe for eyelashes and brows too); neem; rosemary essential oil
lip balm	natural, vegan, cruelty-free versions in limited or compostable packaging; homemade versions; shea butter
lotions and creams	lotion bars; homemade body butter; simple oils like jojoba; minimally packaged, compostable, cruelty-free skincare
makeup-removing wipes	reusable washcloths
mouthwash	salt gargle; water mixed with spearmint, cinnamon, or peppermint essential oils; witch hazel
nail polish and remover	5-, 7-, 8-, and 9-free (meaning formulas are free from potentially harmful ingredients like formaldehyde, toluene, dibutyl phthalate, and more), vegan, cruelty-free versions; soy-based remover; reusable buffers that impart shine sans polish, allowing your nails to breathe
nasal spray	neti pot
plastic toothbrush	compostable bamboo toothbrush

rubber bands	cotton hair bands; reusable hairpins
shampoo	solid shampoo bar; cruelty-free, vegan versions; castile soap; apple cider vinegar and baking soda
shaving cream	shaving bar and cruelty-free shaving brush; castile soap
toothpaste	minimally packaged, cruelty-free, and vegan versions; homemade toothpastes and powders; baking soda
tooth whiteners	activated charcoal powder; certain clay powders
zit cream	tea tree or lavender essential oil

CRIMSON WAVE

It's estimated that the average gal will use ninety-six hundred tampons and pads in her lifetime. And we all know that those items can have loads of associated waste (hello, boxes, wrappers, and applicators) and creepy additives (pesticides, carcinogens, rayon, and plastics).[vii] The good news is that there are plenty of sustainable options that work with your lifestyle and comfort level. If you're an outside-the-bod lady, you may like reusable (washable, so don't freak) pads and period panties. If you're more of an inside-job gal, a reusable menstrual cup (it's literally like a silicone chalice for your vagine) could be for you. The cup is my personal favorite, though it has a bit of a learning curve and is not for those who are spooked by their own anatomy (you really need to get up in there to get it right the first few times). Whatever your preference, these options can be reused for many years, save an estimated $200-plus per year, and reduce chemicals in your lady parts, waste in landfills, and the amount of awkward interactions with prepubescent cashiers who sweat bullets ringing up your jumbo box of tampons and thinking about you bleeding monthly.[viii]

DIY BEAUTY AND GROOMING RECIPES FOR PYTs

DEWY MAKEUP-
REMOVING CLEANSER

Whisks the day away without tugging on your gorg skin

Hi, I'm really pale. I also have fussy, dry, sensitive skin that wigs out whenever it feels like it. Then there was a time when I used to wear a shit ton of makeup (like, high school production of *Phantom of the Opera*-level makeup), and removing that mask was a beast. Foaming cleansers did the job, but they made my skin tight and sad. This cleanser, however, is cushiony and calming, and it removes even stubborn eye makeup. If you're not into ripping your skin to shreds as you remove daily impurities and grime, grab a washcloth and give this a whirl. Bonus: You can use this as a body and facial moisturizer too. When I travel I often just bring a small bottle of this, and I'm good to go.

INGREDIENTS

¼ cup sweet almond oil

¼ cup jojoba oil

1 tablespoon castor oil

5–8 drops lavender essential oil

6 drops geranium essential oil, optional

TOOLS

Repurposed glass bottle and dropper/lid

Reusable washcloth

Put all the ingredients in a bottle (if your skin is very sensitive, skip the essential oils), then do like the Cars and shake it up. When you're ready to use it, place a silver dollar's worth in your palm, and rub gently on your dry face (makeup and all), concentrating on areas that have harder-to-remove makeup. Add more if necessary, and once your face is properly covered and rubbed (someone's gonna snatch that as a porn title, I swear), wet a washcloth with warm water, wring it out, and place it over your face for 10 seconds. Then gently wipe your face with the washcloth until the washcloth comes up clean. Your skin will feel cleansed but not stripped, with a pleasant leftover dewiness.

DECLARATION OF INDEPENDENCE
DRY SHAMPOO

Four score and seven days ago, you washed your hair

Adding to the mounting allure established throughout this book, I should also tell you that I don't wash my hair every day. And neither should you. We hold these truths to be self-evident that you can go days without washing your hair and still have friends. But if I'm really real with you, by the end of the workweek, I've used so much of this dry shampoo that I'm like a low-key founding father signing the Declaration of Independence—powdered wig excellence. It doesn't look it, though, because this recipe is dope, smells great, and means you don't need to spend big bucks on basically the same ingredients in better packaging (unless you want to). Yes, you can liberate yourself from the shackles of the shower and bodify next-day styles with a sprinkle. In grand *MacGyver* fashion, the lighter hair recipe also multitasks as a prevacuum freshener for rugs; a deodorizing sprinkle for sweaty, smelly shoes; body powder to prevent inner-thigh chafe; and underarm deodorant in a pinch. If that ain't modern-day convenience, I don't know what is.

INGREDIENTS

2 teaspoons kaolin clay

3 tablespoons cornstarch

5–10 drops rosemary and lavender essential oils

For darker hair: Add 2 teaspoons cocoa powder,
(or more to get the right color)

TOOLS

Repurposed glass spice bottle and shaker top

For a fine powder, put all of the dry ingredients in a high-speed blender. Once it's nicely mixed, add the essential oils while the blender is set on low. If you have darker hair, add cocoa powder as needed to achieve your desired color. (You can also experiment with adding cinnamon or activated charcoal to achieve the right tint that complements your lustrous locks.) Once you've gotten a mix you're happy with, decant it into the glass bottle, and use whenever. I like to sprinkle this into my bare hands and work it into my roots, but others dig using a fluffy powder brush for more precise application.

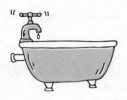

SOAK AWAY THE SICKIES BATH

Cue the C+C Music Factory,
because this bath is gonna make you sweat

Whether you're down with a cold or the flu, can't seem to get warm enough because it's -3°F, or just feel rundown from work and general debauchery, this bath will get you back on track. Packed with ingredients that detoxify, relax your muscles, and give your sinuses some aromatic relief, this magical potion will have you feeling mighty toasty and ready for a restorative good night's sleep.

INGREDIENTS

3 tablespoons ground ginger

¼ cup ground mustard seed

¼ cup baking soda

1 cup Epsom salts

5–10 drops rosemary essential oil

5 drops tea tree oil

The prep on this is dead simple, which is good because I usually make it when I feel like I'm about to ralph: Run a warm bath, mix these ingredients in, submerge thyself, and soak. Because these ingredients can encourage a lot of sweatin', be sure you're drinking plenty of water before and after. Emerge from the tub a new person, ready to be swaddled in cozy pjs and tucked into bed.

QUICK HITS
IN THE MIRROR

Whether you're a makeup maven or an ardent minimalist, these five-minute tips will get you one step closer to liking that sustainable human looking back at you in the mirror.

- Take a peek at your grooming or beauty routine. Do any of the products bear cruelty-free, vegan, or organic symbols? If not, make a vow to replace them with kinder and conscious options when it's time to refill.

- Using the chart on page 222, see if any of the items you currently use can be easily swapped for more sustainable options. And then do just that. A super-painless start? Swap your plastic tooth-brush for a mostly compostable bamboo version, and flash those pearly whites.

- Do the Give a Shit Beauty Fast on page 219. Just do it. Do it now.

- Research cruelty-free and vegan companies and products. Have fun with this! If you're going to online shop and go down a rabbit hole, you may as well do so for goodies that are kinder to, well, rabbits.

- Make your version of my homemade air freshener. Then, spray it around your entire home, dance in the spritz, breathe deeply, and feel happy that you've officially cleared the air sans chemical nasties.

- Love yourself. This may sound hella silly, but living better with less starts with believing that you, with all your so-called blemishes, cellulite, thin hair, and weird cuticles (points to self) are enough. Once you've got that down, you won't be as susceptible to the ads designed to shame us into buying exploitative shit we simply don't need.

Give a Shit:

In the Wild

Y ou've made it this far, which means you're totally crushing this whole "giving a shit" thing. If you're amped about your new habits (as you should be), get excited, because here's where I show you how to take them to the streets, because I know shit-givers are never cooped up—you've got places to be, paper to chase, pipelines to protest, #resist memes to make, and people to dazzle. This chapter will show you how to live a public life commensurate with your eco-values and inspire others to be equally as dope (in a nonobnoxious, more by shining-example kind of way).

NO EXCUSE FOR SINGLE USE

If you've read this far and are still not familiar with the importance of being less trashy, allow me to issue the sleeper hold: Americans create almost four and a half pounds of trash per person per day (that's like carrying around a thirty-plus-pound weight each week), a 169 percent increase from our waste creation in 1960.[1] We can thank many things for this skyrocketing phenomenon: an increased national focus on convenience, busier lives, and the general accessibility of throwaway options. Fortunately, it's super easy to avoid disposables in the wild. Whether it's your morning coffee or evening cocktail(s), building a chic, sleek, and totally essential arsenal of reusable swag will help you refuse that refuse and look like a sustainability siren.

The most common excuse for not using the reusable accoutrements we have at home is because . . . those items are at home. If you pack a cute, portable, sustainable kit with you on the daily, you're more likely to refuse disposables when it counts. Although it may sound painfully hipster (punch me now), I pack a glass Mason jar and lid, bamboo cutlery, a cloth napkin, lightweight reusable shopping bag, and a stainless-steel tiffin (a fancy word for a metal to-go container that usually stacks and looks hella cool) with me pretty much at all times. The bundle doesn't add much weight, but it saves me from having to live that garbage life. Plus, at the risk of sounding like a bourgeoisie bastard, these accoutrements make dining, even at the shadiest establishment (like the bus—no shame), feel like a real, grown-up occasion worth savoring.

Many coffee and tea joints, like Starbucks and Peet's, will give you a discount if you BYO cup. And if your local establishment doesn't incentivize bringing your own, use your words and encourage them to do so. Although coffee biggie Starbucks has been offering customers a BYO discount since 1985, 2010 efforts to publicize and incentivize the reusable program resulted in a 55 percent increase in peeps bringing their own, sparing an estimated 1.5 million pounds of paper from landfills.[2] The moral of the story? A BYO program doesn't just offset supply costs for businesses; it also creates positive momentum in consumer habits.

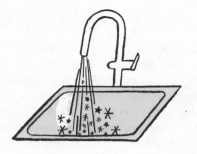

BULLSHIT IN A BOTTLE

You know what's freaking incredible? We live in a country where pretty much everywhere you go, you can flip a handle and get clean, potable water immediately FOR FREE. Isn't that wonderful? And when you consider how much people in developing and compromised areas struggle to get access to safe drinking water, it seems extra silly that we'd eschew our magical home-based Chalice Wells to drop $6 on wasteful bottled water. And let's talk about bottled water for a second, because it's a hot-button issue. Individually the average American uses 167 disposable water bottles each year (but recycles only 20 percent. Bummer). Collectively Americans use about 50 billion plastic water bottles every freaking year, 38 billion of which end up in landfills. This bananas demand for bottled water uses more than 17 million barrels of oil (enough to fuel 1.3 million cars) and enough energy to power 190,000 homes. Not only are these bad boys a major problem for the planet, they're also hella expensive. If you're getting your recommended eight glasses a day from disposable bottles, you could be paying an estimated $1,400 each year, a stark contrast when you consider that the same amount from the tap is around 50 cents, minus the harmful polyethylene terephthalate (PET). So if you make one switch today, let is be lessening your consumption of bottled water (and bottled anything, really).[i]

This shit is really easy to do, guys. Bring your own reusable water bottle wherever you go. You'll save big bucks while also lessening reliance on disposables. If you're traveling, pack an empty reusable bottle in your carry-on and fill it up when you're through security. Voilà! You've just avoided having to pay $10 for a bottle of H_2O.

SASHAY AWAY, STRAWS!

This may seem small because, well, straws are kind of small, but it's an easy place to start, mostly because those cylindrical suckers are freaking EVERYWHERE. And although these sippers may keep your lipstick pristine, most of the five hundred million straws Americans use every freaking day cannot be recycled (they're often too lightweight to make it through the recycling sorter) and, if they don't spend thousands of years in a landfill, make their way into waterways, choking wildlife.[ii] Straws are among the top-ten most prevalent items found during beach cleanups, and an estimated 71 percent of seabirds and 30 percent of turtles have been found with plastics in their stomachs, half of whom die.[iii] I don't know about you, but I really liked the book Jonathan Livingston Seagull *as a kid, and turtles are cool as fuck. We can do better, don't ya think?*

The solution here is simple: stop sucking (also the hashtag for the global campaign launched by heartthrob Adrian Grenier to rid oceans of plastic straws). When you're out at dinner or drinks, ask for no straw. Heck, it could be a great conversation starter with your date or that smoldering specimen sitting next to you at the bar (this actually happened to me once and was magical). And if you're a die-hard user or need one for medical or accessibility reasons, consider packing your own reusable glass or stainless-steel version.

Progress, Not Perfection

If you're caught without your kit, do the best you can by considering these lower-waste approaches:

Beverages: Can you pause for a few minutes and enjoy your drink at the shop in one of their cups or mugs? If a coffee break isn't possible and you're on the move, you'll need a cup, but do you need a lid, straw, sleeve, caddy, or those totally confounding plastic things that plug up the lid's sipping hole? Most likely not. Skip the nonessentials and sip away.

Snack stops: Sometimes you just need a treat on the fly. And for those times, consider whether you really need the paper sleeve, napkins, or container. I've gotten the charming rep at my local bakery as the girl who asks the cashier to "just put the cookie in my hand," and you too can be just as beguiling.

Leftovers: Inquire about the most eco-friendly option for packin' it up. Foil, paper, and even napkins work well for dry things. Reusable or recyclable containers are always better than nonrecyclable plastics and Styrofoam (ughhh, Styrofoam). And for the love of all that's holy, skip the plastic bag to carry it all or go for a paper (read: recyclable) version.

Delivery: I've been there: It's blizzarding, your cupboards are as bare as Mother Hubbard's, and only the Ethiopian place across town will make you feel human again. Many places and food-ordering apps will happily accommodate you specifying no cutlery, napkins, bags, mints, wet wipes, sauce packets, religious pamphlets, romance novels, and whatever else they usually throw in there.

Shopping: Even shopping till you drop (per the Give a Shit ethical parameters, obvs) can be done without creating unnecessary waste. Ask for no receipt or an electronic version upfront. Often, before you even know what's happening, a sales associate will start swaddling even nonfragile or gift purchases in tissue paper, bows, stickers, ribbons, bags, and other unnecessary shit, so start the transaction by saying you won't be needing that noise. And because many of us already carry enormous bags on the daily, drive cars, and/or have these remarkable things called hands expressly designed to carry shit, try using those to tote your purchases instead of taking the cashier up on disposable bags. Yes, you can fit a mascara in your purse, girl. Move some shit around. I believe in you.

Places that won't let you BYO: Plans to sneak roasted chickpeas and a Mason jar full of whiskey into the movie theater been foiled? Been there. Concert or baseball game won't allow you to fill up your own cup? Shit happens. Make the least wasteful selections possible, focusing on reuse, recyclability, or rot-ability (hint: the easiest way to do all three is to just avoid plastic as much as possible), and party on.

These strategies don't require perfection, just thoughtfulness about what you actually need in each situation.

WORK, WORK, WORK, WORK, WORK

Although some folks have work-from-home or travel-all-the-time arrangements, many of us do the nine-to-five-ish grind at an office. No matter your occupational situation, there are plenty of ways to stay true to giving a shit without being a fussy, judgmental dickhead. When I first got into this way of life, I was working at a company that never recycled. So I would stay later and sift through the trash, salvaging recyclables and hauling them to the nearest receptacle. This doesn't just make me totally dateable, it also annoyed the hell out of our office manager, who felt I was trying to usurp her nonexistent recycling duties—and we all know how scorned office managers can make your work life a living hell. So I did what any fearful twentysomething would do—I issued my mea culpa in

the form of a pecan pie and a succulent plant. And after she softened (bitch loved pecans), I asked her if she'd help me develop an
in-house office recycling program. She agreed, and we ended up
becoming a jolly good green team, instituting cool stuff like in-of-
fice composting and animal shelter volunteering days. Sure, some
people, like naysayer Mark, who would take credit for other people's work and chew with his mouth open, hated the new recycling
regime for a second, and then folks got really, almost weirdly into it.

These changes are even easier to institute when you're the
head honcho. If you own a company or oversee an office, by golly,
nothing says "I'm not a regular boss, I'm a cool boss" like being at
the forefront of workplace sustainability. American offices are really

PACK IT UP

There was a time when bringing your lunch was considered decidedly uncool
and could even get you beat up. Those times, thankfully, are over (well, at
least in the office realm and, I hope, in schools too), and lunch bringing is
now a sign that someone kind of has their act together. Here's some truth:
lunchtime is the trashiest time in the American day, and it's not because
many of us are skimming celebrity gossip on our breaks. Here's the deal:
approximately one-third of all food is wasted at the retail and consumer
levels, and that means establishments where we dine and take out, which
happens most often during lunchtime. Even in relatively small districts like
Minneapolis, which has about 35,717 students, school cafeterias alone can
create 483,520 pounds of waste per day (that's 13.5 pounds of trash per
day, per pupil).[iv] When done right, packing your lunch has been shown to
cut down on waste, keep people healthier, and save money.

Start small, and commit to bringing your lunch two to three times a
week (find make-ahead recipes in the Kitchen section that make this easy
peasy), and I promise you'll get so into that healthy-feeling, money-saving,
lunch-bringing zone that you'll want to do it all the time. Trust.

wasteful places. According to the EPA, up to 45 percent of municipal waste is generated in the workplace.[3] A McKinsey Global Institute study showed an uptick in executives aligning sustainability with other business goals because greener workplaces are simply good business, generating significant cost savings, increased worker productivity (by 16 percent, in some cases), and enhanced public perception (an estimated one-third of consumers prefer sustainable brands).[4] In addition to the nifty eco-techniques laid out in the home office section, here are some ideas that will keep your office life aligned with giving a shit:

Have a reusable kit at your desk: A water bottle or glass, coffee mug, plate, bowl, cutlery, and a cloth napkin tucked neatly in your desk drawer will eliminate the need for any typical office waste culprits. Plus, it makes you look like a refined son of a bitch. I also keep a silicone reusable bag with me so I can take food scraps home to compost, but consider that extra credit if you're just getting started.

Join or start a green team: This may sound lame, but I would posit that a team dedicated to workplace sustainability is just as cool as that intramural office kickball team, with way less likelihood of seeing your boss in short-shorts. Mobilizing and empowering your coworkers to crowdsource and enact sustainable processes increases organizational buy-in (strength in numbers, people). Make sure you run this by any other stakeholders who would appreciate involvement or a heads-up. And, if you need any more incentive to get people to adopt and join, bill it as a one-stop-shop for cost savings, community building, and professional development (because it is!).

Suggest integrating sustainability more officially: Like into your yearly review or the company's annual report. Major brands such as Apple, Walmart, Nike, and almost every other Fortune 500 company have sustainability metrics built into their core values and business goals, so come on, all the cool kids are doing it.[5]

Ditch the disposables: For smaller offices it's especially easy to hit up a resale shop and buy some charmingly mismatched mugs (I have one from the thrift store that says "Bikini Inspector"), plates, and other kitchen items and eschew disposables. Yes, you'll have to remind people that the office manager is not their mom and that they need to wash their fucking dishes, but you'll reduce trash and save the office dough (that can then be channeled into karaoke happy hours). Moreover, affordable, sustainable office supply options abound, and implementing them is sometimes as simple as chatting with the person who does the purchasing. Do it. I currently work at a very large Fortune 500 company, and a five-minute hallway chat with our supplies buyer resulted in a quick switch to buying recyclable cutlery. If your office is in need of new furnishings, secondhand is a great way to go that also means your graphic design department can look like a rad 1990s personal injury law office. You're welcome in advance.

Institute recycling and composting: Just as you did in your own home, you can make recycling and composting easy and almost automatic at the office with subscription pick-up and drop-off services. Again, talk to your office or building manager, and you might be surprised how easy this is to implement: you already have a daily UPS pickup, so how hard could it be to add a daily compost grab?

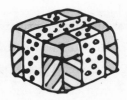

Gift green: When it's time to give your coworkers or clients gifts, consider giving them something thoughtful (like an experience gift) or reusable (like a cool travel mug or mini French press). Sometimes eco-friendly gifts are the best peer pressure gateway drug for someone who's interested in giving a shit but not quite motivated to start by themselves. Many years ago a politician client would see me ordering vegan options and bringing my little Mason jar whenever we traveled together, and remarked, "I should do that. I'm just too busy to remember." So for the holidays I gifted him and his wife dinner at an amazing plant-based restaurant (ahem, Vedge in Philadelphia. Go. Now.) and a boss-looking stainless-steel water bottle. When I caught up with him years later, after I'd transitioned careers, he still had that bottle with him and called it "old faithful." Brings a tear to my eye.

Share your passion: Yes, I was that kid who got ridiculously amped about talking about my hermit crab at show-and-tell. I also know that you've probably sat through work-mandated "Lunch and Learns" that make you want to build a time machine and reclaim those fifty minutes of soggy sandwiches and spreadsheets. If you're passionate and well versed about sustainable living (which, after reading this, you totes are) and you've got a hunch that your coworkers might share that enthusiasm, sing that shit loud and proud and give a presentation on the importance of sustainable shifts, bring in a dope vegan meal, or screen an eco-documentary. (And, conversely, genuinely show enthusiasm for and interest in your coworkers' initiatives. No one's gonna listen to or care about your shit if you're a self-absorbed tool.)

Know (and influence) the policies: If your company has a work-from-home policy, by golly, use it. And if they don't, make the case for one (increased productivity, lower overhead, reduced waste and travel emissions). Moreover, many companies will match charitable giving, which can give your donations to sustainability-minded organizations extra zing, so ensure you're maximizing those.

LOVE, MARRIAGE, AND THE BABY CARRIAGE

Interpersonal relationships can be tricky, especially when smooching is involved. Here are a few tips for navigating romantic waters whilst keeping your newly minted eco–street cred fresh to till-death-do-you-part.

Dating

Whether you're in the market for a booty call or a go-the-distance relationship, it's always nice to be with someone who gets you. Now, I totally understand you might be panicking, thinking, *This dating shit is hard enough as it is, and now I have a somewhat not-as-mainstream (but super rad) lifestyle added to the mix?* Never fear! Here I am to be your wing woman:

Expand your circle: Hey, you're probably a bit more into sustainability and caring about animals and the planet now, right?

Awesome. There are communities of people who are in the same headspace. Get active volunteering, protesting, going to meet-ups, and even exploring some of the newer online dating sites for plant-based and sustainability-minded singles (though, admittedly, I haven't tried 'em so I can't speak to them in detail).

Be upfront: For years I would be demure about the fact that I was into animal rights because I worried that potential partners would find it deterrent. And, to be totally frank, some did. However, more suitors than not were attracted to my passion. Some even adopted a vegetarian lifestyle or, long after our rendezvous fizzled, still pop in to tell me they buy cruelty-free soap. But more importantly I knew I was being true to me. Do you really want to hide a passionate part of yourself or be with someone who doesn't respect your values and choices? Didn't think so. So let your eco-freak flag fly on those dating profiles or in those clandestine bar conversations. Listen, shit-giver, your penguin is out there (if that's what you want), and said person will be drawn to and respect that fire in your belly. After all, someone who has gusto, whether it's about sustainability or quilt-ing, is a hell of a lot more interesting than someone who doesn't give a shit about anything.

But be cool: This should go without saying, but not everyone comes out of the womb with your same habits and beliefs. Yes, have your boundaries and convictions, but be open to respectful and inquisi-tive dialogue (which can be way attractive, BTW), and if someone isn't a fit or insults that which you hold most dear, well, bye, Felicia.

Make it an adventure: Boo thang's never been to a vegetarian restaurant? Bae's never met a cow up close? Explore together! Try out a new-to-you, plant-forward cuisine, take a trip to an animal sanctuary, or volunteer for a beach cleanup. Your curiosity and resolve will strengthen along with your bond. Besides, caring and compassion are sexy. Speaking of which...

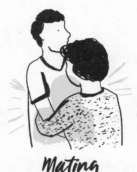

Mating

Don't worry: I'm not going to get awkward about this, but because we're all adults and are probably rendered equally helpless when we hear a Keith Sweat song, I'm going to lay down some ways you can make getting busy greener. Let me preface: I am not a medical professional—it's your body, so if any of these sound interesting to you, consult your physician first. I'll also posit that preventing unwanted pregnancies, as we'll cover a few sections down, is one of the most eco-friendly things you can do, so if an occasional condom wrapper or pill package makes its way into the trash can because you're being diligent, I say good on you. That said, there are some interesting innovations in the realm of more sustainable sexin' that may strike your fancy.

Just the tips: Again, I'm not a doctor. I am, however, an appreciator of the many freedoms made possible by accessible birth control. That said, some studies have shown that an unfortunate side effect of the Pill is residual synthetic hormones in our drinking water.[6] If you're not into that or the attendant packaging waste, consider an IUD, which comes in hormone and nonhormone versions, sets up shop in your uterus for up to ten years, and is extremely effective (99.2 percent).[7] If something semipermanent isn't your bag, barrier methods like removable diaphragms, cervical caps, and condoms have you (literally) covered with fewer negative effects on your ecosystem.

If you're with a trusted partner/s and don't require STD protection (though if you've ever watched *Maury*, you know it's a swell idea just in case . . .), many peeps like to get back to basics with the rhythm method, which involves a combination of diligently track-

WRAP IT UP

Allow me to get all college RA, minus the banana demo, and talk condoms for a minute. You have three options when it comes to rubbers (not all of which are rubber, BTW), and they each boast varying degrees of effectiveness and eco-impact.

* *Lambskin: Biodegradable, but do not protect against STDs—and they're lambskin, which I personally do not want in my magical vagina.*

* *Latex: Protects against STDs but cannot be recycled. However, if they're 100 percent pure latex, will biodegrade over time. I dig brands like Sustain, which are fair trade (child labor is often used to source rubber), FSC certified, cruelty-free, vegan (dairy by-products like casein are often used in conventional condoms), and have limited and, whenever possible, recyclable packaging.*

* *Polyurethane: Protects against STDs but are essentially plastic and, thus, cannot be recycled and won't biodegrade.*

Also, I hope this goes without saying, but although reuse is a cornerstone of the Give a Shit lifestyle, please, for Pete's sake, do not go all 1800s courtesan and try to reuse condoms. After doing the deed, wrap condoms in toilet paper and deposit in the garbage so municipal workers don't have to handle a small bag full of your sexual fluids.

ing your cycle and temperature, withdrawal, and barrier method use during fertile days. Effectiveness varies from 76 to 88 percent, but many women note lack of side effects commonly associated with hormonal birth control and the attendant feeling of being more "in touch" with their bodies.[8] Whatever you're opting for, tracking your cycle can give you a newfound appreciation for how freaking rad your reproductive system is, so if that sounds fun, peep apps like Clue and Natural Cycles. And if you're very freaking sure you do not wish to procreate at all or anymore, sterilization is the most long-term and sustainable option. It's also pretty much permanent, so don't go getting wasted and undergo elective sterilization like you would a spur-of-the-moment tattoo. As with any decision involving your body, consider your options and chat with a doc about what makes sense for you.

Family Matters

I know this is going to be a sensitive topic, but I cannot talk about lessening environmental burden without at least addressing family planning, more commonly known (and vilified) as population control. Now, don't get me wrong: this isn't an affront to families or littles—kids are freaking awesome. They are also people, and as we know, people generally suck up resources. A study of developed countries from Lund University in Sweden found that having one fewer child reduced 58.6 tons of CO_2 emissions per year.[9] We're currently around 7.5 billion peeps, and the UN predicts that, at this rate, we'll hit about 9.7 billion people by 2050.[10] If our planet is suffering this much under the resource burden of our current population, what do you think it'll be like with 30 percent more people?

Before you brand me the "Baby Shower Bummer," I simply want to posit some more sustainable alternatives to going full-on *21 Kids and Counting.*

Education and resources for women: Education on and access to family planning for *every* woman are important tenets of a sustainable future. Sure, knowing your personal birth control options and thinking before you have a kid are always good ideas, but advocating for equitable family planning education and resources for people—especially women—around the world is a statistically proven way to stem unwanted births, fetal mortality, and complications like economic strain and societal stigmas that arise from unplanned parenthood, as well as to support global reproductive health and economic security. The Intergovernmental Panel on Climate Change (IPCC) included access to reproductive health services, especially for women in developing countries, as an important factor for reducing greenhouse gasses in its 2014 synthesis.[11]

General education for women is also an important factor in reducing unwanted births, infant mortality, child marriages, disease transmissions, and shoring up socioeconomic mobility and resilience in natural disasters (which we know are likely to affect lower-lying, developing countries first as a result of climate change). According to the Brookings Institution, "the difference between a woman with no schooling and a woman with twelve years of schooling is four to five children," which is especially evident in areas where females have little access to education and that also have skyrocketing populations.[12] So find organizations doing culturally sensitive, evidence-based female empowerment work in underserved areas, and support the hell out of them—ideologically, fiscally, and through volunteering.

Fostering and adoption: When I was about eight years old, I used to stay up late at night watching infomercials because they're incredible. After seeing a "Sponsor a Child" ad, I raced into my sleeping parents' bedroom and begged them to do so, thinking that said child would arrive the next day and be my new bro or sis. My parents groggily agreed, and I stayed up all night, excited as fuck, thinking I was getting a sibling. You can imagine my despair when I was gently informed the next morning that that wasn't how that stuff works. That disenchantment aside, my reverence for adoption abided, and later I became a social worker and child welfare adviser for two governors. Let me tell you: adoption is always dope, but the kiddos in the state systems are freaking incredible and yet grossly overlooked. According to the most recent federal data, there are currently more than one hundred thousand youth waiting to be adopted in the United States, and these kids move an average of seven times while in care.[13] SEVEN TIMES. I don't even like to move my car when it snows. That's a lot of kids who would love to have a consistent home and become part of a family.

I firmly believe that family is more than just blood and biology, so if you're earnest about being a parent or building your family, consider fostering or adoption. And while you're at it, why not look into adopting differently abled, multiracial, and older youth or sibling groups? Those cohorts are often passed over for younger kids and account for many of the more than twenty thousand youth who "age out" of the system each year. These individuals essentially grow up and eventually out of the system around eighteen to twenty-one years of age, depending on the state, without being adopted. With few avenues of support or consistent connections, youth who age out are fourteen times more likely to not complete college and disproportionately experience homelessness (25 percent), unemployment (47 percent), and incarceration (29 percent), among other challenges.[14] Hi, do you remember what you were like when you were eighteen years old? Could you make it on your own with no reliable contacts or supports? Dude, I could barely wear nonpajama pants in public. Imperfect as you think you are, I guarantee you'd be a welcomed help to an older youth on the precipice of adulthood.

Getting Hitched

Weddings are my favorite for two reasons: (1) the joining together of two peeps in love and (2) the high likelihood that I'll get to dance the Macarena. But nuptial celebrations have a dark side, and no, I don't mean Grandma Kiki's cleavage. In addition to the ever-skyrocketing cost of the average American wedding ($35,329 in 2015), each "I do" produces four hundred to six hundred pounds

PUT A RING ON IT

Decades of strategic marketing campaigns have rendered Americans obsessed with diamond engagement rings. The frenzy has become so ingrained in the fabric of Western courtship that there are even engagement ring emporiums and social mores insisting that gents spend three months' salary to prove their love. But behind the sparkles, those precious minerals and gems are often mined by exploited people, including children, in war-torn areas. If you've ever seen Blood Diamond (and weren't too distracted by Leo's chiseled profile), you know what I'm talking about. Consider vintage or secondhand baubles for your nuptials (or any fine jewelry purchase), and if you need new, insist on conflict-free or synthetic stones, recycled precious metals, and local craftsmanship whenever possible.

early 1920s

of garbage and sixty-six tons of carbon dioxide—that's the equivalent of the emissions four to five people create in an entire year.[15] And because there are about 2.3 million weddings annually in the United States and only two of those are Kim Kardashian's, that's a lot of waste, guys. Food, flowers, decorations, favors, elaborate invitations—all that stuff requires significant production, travel, and disposal resources. Now, an entire book could be dedicated to eco-conscious celebrations, but here are a few ideas that can make your nuptials more responsible:

Invitations: Cut down on paper waste by doing electronic invitations and save-the-dates, or opt for seed paper, which can be planted. And go the extra mile to avoid paper waste by asking guests to either not wrap gifts or be that way awesome couple who doesn't have a registry of knick-knacks at all.

Guests: You're super tight with four hundred people? I don't buy it. If you can, pare down your list to the really important attendees. After all, more people = more resources.

Location: Choose a location that's beautiful all by itself (hi, nature!) to reduce décor needs. If it's an indoor fête, consider Leadership in Energy and Environmental Design (LEED)-certified spaces for more responsible energy consumption.

Food: The average meal travels fifteen hundred freaking miles.[16] One meal! When it comes to feeding a bevy of relatives, sourcing locally beats serving organic. Explore more homegrown options, and opt for plant-based menus so you spare the animals whilst celebrating your union.[17]

Booze: Of course your wedding needs alcohol. Consider nearby breweries, distilleries, and vineyards to reduce transportation emissions. People will still get jolly with the added bonus of sampling some local flavor. Win-win.

Flowers: My first job was in a flower shop, and I'm a real sucker for blooms. But there's a seedy underbelly to these beauties. Most flowers are imported from countries like Kenya, Vietnam, and Ecuador, where employees live in poverty, can earn as little as $1 for a twelve-hour day, and are exposed to dangerous chemicals. Sounds romantic, right? If you must have flora, consider locally sourced and in-season potted plants and flowers. They make nice gifts, are easy to rehome, and can be composted.

Balloons: Look, I loved the movie *Up!* as much as anyone, but balloons, magical as they may seem, kinda blow. In the grand rule of gravity, what goes up must come down, and balloons of all types eventually come back to earth as—you guessed it—litter. Latex and Mylar balloons take forever to break down and confuse the hell out of land and sea animals, who either get tangled in or ingest them thinking they're colorful tasty things, thereby blocking their digestive system so they slowly starve to death.[18] I know, this is a major drag, but you can still do fun, commemorative shit, like throwing wildflower seeds or petals, that don't involve hurling actual trash into the air.

Décor: Consider repurposed or upcycled décor. If you are turning your nose up at this, I have two words for you: Mason jars, which can be found secondhand for a song.

Favors: Skip them and make donations instead. Honestly, no one wants salt and pepper shakers bearing your likenesses. Someone had to tell you.

Clothing: Secondhand and vintage dresses and suits are cool as hell, gentler on the earth, and way easier on your wallet. And who mandated that bridal parties needed to look like the Lawrence Welk dancers? Do your wedding how you want, but if matchy-matchy friends aren't your thing, eschew the wasteful new duds for resale scores or simple items you probably already own.

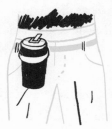

MOVIN' AND SHAKIN'

As mentioned, shit-givers never stay still. We're doing big things, and sometimes those things require us to get all John Candy and hop a plane, train, or automobile. Here's how you can make every-day transit and travel more sustainable, at least until teleportation becomes a reality.

Around Town

When I was a teen, I'd stupidly and regularly pray for two things: (1) to not be the last girl in school to get my period (I was) and (2) an apple-green Dodge Neon (never happened). You see, in the large swath of car-obsessed land known as Texas, if you didn't have wheels, you basically weren't going anywhere without your parents. Not so coincidentally, thanks to my love of fast food (see recipe homage to Arby's on page 168) and activity level equivalent to that of a mall cop I was a pretty husky kid. It wasn't until I went to college in a more navigable-by-foot city that I was introduced to the magic of greener, leaner public transit options. Now, if this were a nineties teen movie, I'd have instantly morphed into svelte, man-trap Ashlee upon setting foot in Boston, removing my glasses, and unfurling my ponytail. That didn't quite happen, but I did drop some LBs while gaining a deep appreciation for the eco-friendly magic of trains, buses, and bikes.

Car-ried away: My experience isn't terribly unique. The United States boasts more cars than licensed drivers, and those cars and trucks account for 20 percent of all US emissions, with each gallon of gas causing twenty-four pounds of CO_2 emissions.[19] I'm no rocket scientist, guys, but do you think the fact that 66 percent of Americans are overweight or obese is pure coincidence?[20] This car crowding means that the average American commuter spends forty-two hours and $960 a year just sitting in (and swearing at) traffic.[21] Recent studies suggest that living car-free is a potent step in tackling climate change, sparing 2.4 tons of carbon dioxide each year.[22] If, however, you desperately need a car for work or picking up chicks, keep what you've got in good repair and drive it sparingly. If you're in the market for new wheels, consider low-emission hybrid and no-emission electric versions. If you need a car less frequently, look into car shares, short-term rentals, and carpooling.

Come on, ride the train: Or bus. Or bike. Park the car, and give one of the 150 metro systems worldwide, countless buses and trolleys, and one thousand global bike-share programs a spin.[23] And if those options aren't readily available in your area, kick-push a skateboard, steal the neighbor kid's tricycle (kidding), wheel your chair around town like a bat out of hell, or take a freaking walk.

Going the Distance

Sometimes life calls us to places where planes are our only feasible mode of transit. The aviation industry accounts for about 2 percent of the world's emissions, with a single round-trip coach ticket from New York to San Francisco creating two metric tons of carbon dioxide.[24] Employing thoughtful strategies before takeoff and after landing can help you straighten the fuck up and fly right.

Offset: If air travel is your only option, consider purchasing offset credits, which, for a nominal fee, supposedly neutralize carbon emissions associated with your trip. I say "supposedly" because offset credits have garnered a lot of criticism (how do we know if the fee is actually being put to use?) as modern-day snake oil. Carriers like Delta and United allow you to calculate and purchase offsets when you book, and third parties like Terrapass let you offset whenever you darn well please.

Book nonstop: Most airplane carbon emissions stem from takeoff and landing, so minimize the amounts of flights it takes to get you from point A to point B.[25] You're welcome for a valid reason to #treatyoself to a trip with no layovers.

Pack light: You'll reduce weight, thereby reducing the plane's energy use (and cutting down on the very real stress associated with schlepping a fifty-pound bag around an airport). Hint: this isn't as much of an issue if you've pared down per chapters 3 and 4.

Ditch disposables: From an electronic ticket, to bringing your own food from home, to passing on in-flight beverage and snack services, every little bit matters.

Fly coach: If you're me, you're thinking, *as if I had a choice*. But, hey, if you're flush enough to fly first class, consider that those larger, heavier seats take up more space and weight and have footprints six times larger than those economy seats.[26] Yes, this means you'll have to huddle among the unwashed masses (me), but you're welcome to sleep on my shoulder, Kanye.

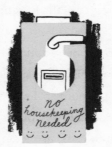

Stay Green

Although the journey is half the fun, temporarily setting up shop at your destination after arduous travel is like an oasis in the desert. Plus, there's something oh so alluring about sprawling in a big, freshly starched bed in a room you never have to clean yourself. That said, let's not go too bananas. Hotels are bastions of bad eco-behaviors, largely because we can become total douchebags when we're on vacation. Because we're finally in a space we don't have to clean, we sometimes feel more inclined to use a billion towels and a bunch of mini-toiletries and expect fresh sheets, turndown service, and a chocolate on our pillow after every nap. Here are some ways to keep giving a shit whilst kicking up your vacay-mode heels.

Book green: Whenever booking your home away from home, use a green booking engine (I like greenhotelworld.com), and seek out LEED-certified buildings and TripAdvisor's Green Leaders Program members.

Pass on housekeeping: Doing so saves laundry-related energy, and nobody really needs twelve clean towels for a two-day stay.[27]

Avoid using mini-toiletries: Those baby bottles of soap are just trash waiting to happen. If you do use some, take them home with you and either reuse the containers or donate them to homeless shelters or organizations like Clean the World, which distributes hotel toiletries to people in areas lacking proper sanitation.

Limit your energy use as you would at home: Hotel stays are hella fun, but they don't merit blasting the television and A/C 24/7.

Share feedback: At the end of your stay, let the establishment know that you either appreciated their green initiatives or you would love to see more.

Skip the rental: Car, that is. Walk, take up on city bikes or hotel bike sharing, use public transit, and, if you must have a set of wheels, opt for electric or hybrid options when available.

Eat neat: Whether you're visiting a nearby town or a far-off destination, getting to sample unique local fare is one of the great joys of travel. It's also one of the greenest things you can do. Explore farmers' markets, support local food artisans, use your reusable arsenal, and find amazing plant-based options anywhere in the world using apps like Happy Cow.

Holidays and Celebrations

People who know me will attest that I'm legit always down to party. And although holidays like Christmas are deemed the most wonderful times of the year, they're also the most wasteful. During this most wasterful wonderland, Americans on average consume 80 percent more food than they do during the rest of the year, spend upward of $1,200 on gifts and decorations (that's more than double what we spent in 2008), and produce 25 percent more trash (about twenty-five million extra tons) from just Thanksgiving to New Year's.[28] Thankfully, a little mindfulness means you can avoid these phenomena and still have a rockin' good time. Also, these strategies can be used for any kind of hearty partying. So, whatever and whenever you're celebrating, consider greening your fête.

Share the wealth: As mentioned before, instead of going out and buying a bunch of new decorations, serving dishes, chocolate fountains, DJ booths, or whatever, beat your local bushes for borrowing and rental options.

Decorations: When I was growing up, we made truly hideous ornaments from homemade dough, garlands from old popcorn, and reused the same janky artificial tree and busted lights for decades. Nowadays some peeps buy everything new each year and actually hire holiday décor professionals to deck their halls. What the fuck? Whatever you celebrate, I'm pretty sure the general ethos is joy, giving back, appreciation, and togetherness. Nowhere have I ever seen a holiday centered on having the best wreaths in the neighborhood. You can embellish your home tastefully with existing décor and repurposed and natural items without spending a fortune (a leaf garland is gorgeous and virtually free). And if your celebration requires a tree, for instance, consider living potted or rentable versions, responsibly recycle the thirty-three million live trees sold each year (at designated drop-off sites), or reuse and repair your artificial versions so they'll stand tall for decades.

Greeting cards: What once was a symbol of true thoughtfulness has morphed into an oft-dreaded landfill pariah. Although color-coordinated family photos and winding narratives about how little Johnny made honor roll this year are touching, after doing time on your mantle for, oh, twenty or so days, most of the 2.65 billion Christmas cards sold each year are chucked. If everyone sent one less card during the holidays, fifty thousand cubic yards of paper would be preserved.[29] So opt for e-cards or emails, and if that's just too millennial for you, show people you really care by picking up the dang phone and giving them a ring dingy. In a day and age when texts are the norm, calling someone to catch up is a deeply genuine way to show you give a shit.

Eat ethically: Holidays aren't celebratory for farmed animals; they're a massacre. Sixty-seven million turkeys are killed every year for Thanksgiving and Christmas alone.[30] As we've established, these creatures feel pain and fear. Celebrate without the suffering by serving sumptuous plant-based cuisine.

Give thoughtfully: I think we've firmly established that we all have enough stuff. Infants won't remember receiving a heap of presents, and what people crave most are adventure, memories, and quality time. Gift loved ones experiences they'll treasure or need, thoughtful secondhand finds, always-adored plants, or go to town making homemade body butters, granola, or spice blends. I'm not suggesting you abstain from gifts, but I do encourage you to simplify your approach. A trending philosophy for kid's gifts is "want, need, wear, read," as in, give them one item they really want (LEGOS), one item they need (compostable toothbrush), something they'll wear (super-dope Transformers mittens), and a book to read (*The Giving Tree*), and this rubric can be applied to damn near anyone. If you're going the gift card route, opt for electronic versions, as most physical gift cards are made from PVC and require special recycling. And if your gift requires batteries, reach for rechargeable.

Wrap responsibly: Giftwrap and shopping bags account for four million tons of holiday trash, much of which cannot be recycled due to additives like glitter and plastic.[31] Preserve surprise and delight responsibly by swathing gifts in repurposed wrappings, newspaper, and reusable cloth options like Japanese furoshiki, and adorn with natural items like herbs, leaves, and recycled ribbons. And once the unveiling is over, save what you can to reuse next year, recycle, or compost. When you need to mail packages, use shipping materials you already have, and go for paper tape, which can be recycled.

PARTIES WITH A PURPOSE

For many folks the singular objective of drunk karaokeing "Semi-Charmed Life" is enough purpose to party. But hey, if you're going to get your peeps together, why not have your gathering give back?

* **Shelter supplies:** Corks, old tees, and other materials can be used to make toys and supplies for lonely animals in shelters. Call your local shelter or rescue for the 411 on what they need and will accept.

* **Cookies for seniors:** Turn the traditional holiday cookie swap on its head by experimenting with tasty plant-based recipes and bringing your creations to lonely seniors. They'll appreciate the thought and company, and your waistline won't miss the sixty-seven pecan sandies you ate out of obligation last year. Check with local senior outreach organizations to learn their regulations on home-baked donations.

* **Homeless care packages:** This is my favorite kind of party. When I couldn't make it home for the holidays, I spent a chilly Christmas with a few other Chicago-bound friends, sipping spiked cider and making these care packages that we then passed out to the homeless. And honestly, despite missing my family, it was the best Christmas of my life because it embodied the true spirit and joy of giving. Have everyone bring their unwanted but still useful gloves, hats, socks, undershirts, toiletries, and bags and purses, and stuff the bags with goodies to create useful care packages that will really brighten someone's day. Some of our packages had perfume and cologne samples, and one female recipient began to cry, saying it had been so long since she'd smelled good and that she was too ashamed to go into a department store and spritz a tester. You never know how something seemingly useless to you can totally transform someone's day and life.

These shindigs embody the spirit of repurposing while also being thoughtful of others. Compassion is a cornerstone of giving a shit, and it feels way better than a two-day hangover anyway (though, far be it from me to stop you from having both).

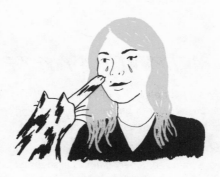

PET PALS

If Harry Potter has taught us anything, it's that your life gets ten times more magical with an animal companion. Not only are animals funny as hell, but research also supports that critters can reduce stress, improve human health and activity levels, increase our social interactions, expose kiddos to important germs to protect against allergy development, and help nurture compassion, responsibility, and respect.[32] My dog not only provides emotional support (she comes running to comfort you if you cry, a gift I have exploited by fake crying one too many times), but she also keeps things interesting by loudly cleaning her crotch the moment company arrives. If all of that sounds just too good to be true and you want one of your own, consider these ethical ways to welcome the furry, feathered, spiky, and scaly into your home.

Adopt, don't shop: Allow me to drop some truth here: what we call a "puppy mill" (cue the Sarah McLachlan song) is just a bad animal-breeding operation left unchecked. And there are a lot of them. You know what else there are a lot of in the United States? Wonderful animals in shelters and rescues. About 6.5 million of 'em each year, actually—1.5 million of whom are euthanized largely due

SUSTAINABLE SUPPLIES

Having an animal pal doesn't need to be a giant waste-creator or strain on your wallet. Pets are a bit like children—we've been told they need shiny, new things, but really, they end up enjoying the box those things come in even more. Explore what your pet needs and what is accessible to you. For me, I've found the following work well:

* **Food:** Pups can safely and healthfully enjoy a vegan diet, so says my and other veterinarians (for cats and other critters, this is debatable), so I buy the biggest bag available so it travels less and recycle the paper packaging, and she's stocked for months like a doomsday prepper.[v]

* **Treats:** Homemade treats are an inexpensive and easy way to use up food waste (like almond meal from making almond milk), and most pet treats can be purchased in bulk with your own bags at farmers' markets and major retailers like Pet Supplies Plus.

* **Toys:** My pup sates her chew fix with ice cubes (cheap, hydrating, and zero cleanup) and naturally-shed antlers. When she's winnowed them down to alarmingly sharp shivs, I toss them in the compost. I also tie together old fabric scraps (from orphaned socks, underwear, and rags) to make tug toys that she really digs. Cats, refined bastards that they are, like toys made from wine corks (a simple Google search yields tons of DIY vids). So drink up!

* **Beds:** My dog's favorite bed is mine, but her next favorite is one I made from an old pillow insert (that otherwise would've headed to the landfill) and a very worn concert tee. When it starts to reek from all her snack hoarding and aforementioned, super-classy crotch cleaning, I throw it in the wash, and it comes out ready to fight another day.

* **Waste removal:** Biodegradable poop bags and litters (pine!) with limited packaging cut down on waste when your buddy answers nature's call.

* **Bathing:** Your pets want to smell like hot garbage. You want to have friends and be able to breathe freely in your home. So sometimes baths need to happen. Keep 'em short, cool, and simple with naturally fragrant castile soap (I use Dr. Bronner's tea tree on my gal).

* **Flea prevention:** Fleas are tenacious bastards that can jump one hundred times their body length, and if your critter catches them, they can make your life miserable and decidedly unsustainable (you have to wash everything all the time, forever and ever amen). Thankfully, essential oils like cedar, lemongrass, and rosemary along with powdery diatomaceous earth can safely rid and sometimes prevent your friend and abode of those unwelcomed guests without harsh chemicals.

to lack of space or homes.[33] Give those guys a hand by fostering or adopting your next best bud instead of buying from a breeder or pet store. More than 120 US cities have banned the selling of dogs and cats at pet stores to encourage adoption because it's just the right thing to do. And if you have your heart set on a purebred, be patient and check out breed-specific rescues. No joke, adopting my dog was the best $65 I ever spent. And I guarantee you'll feel the same way when you mosey over to the shelter and save a life. High-fives!

Spay and neuter: The days of people thinking it's way neat that your dog "accidentally" had puppies are over, man. With so many unwanted and, in turn, euthanized animals languishing in shelters nationwide, intentionally or unintentionally breeding more just ain't cool. I'm gonna sound like Bob Barker at the end of *The Price Is Right*, but be responsible and spay and neuter your pets. Not only will doing so cut down on unwanted critters, but it can also curb aggressive and destructive behaviors. If a fix is out of your budget, there are loads of low- and no-cost options through local shelters and community programs that will snip your furry friends in a jiffy for free. Moreover, if you're in an area replete with feral cats, call Animal Services (PETA also has a helpful 24/7 hotline) and work with authorities to get said critters spayed/neutered and then into an open admission shelter where they can stay safe and warm until they're adopted.

VOLUNTEERING AND ACTIVISM

Whew! You've made it, which means you're basically cooler, more aware, and sexier than you were before you started this book. You're probably also kind of fired up, am I right? If you're ready to dig deep and double-down on your impact, volunteering and activism are natural extensions of walking your talk.

Let's get political: Wherever you live, there's a level of accessible government or leadership. In America we enjoy the beautiful and oft-taken-for-granted gift of being able to vote and actively engage with politics. So although much of this book pivots on individual actions to stem climate change, the world will heal much, much faster if we take action on all levels. Get involved by tracking issues and policies; attending lobby days; offering grassroots or even full-on campaign volunteer support to candidates who give a shit; canvassing and petitioning; staying abreast of current events and research via credible sources; and, for heaven's sakes, exercising your precious right to vote whenever possible. Few things are more annoying than an armchair philosopher who bitches about the state of affairs without ever actually doing anything to help.

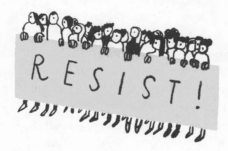

Fight the power: Personal responsibility and political advocacy are crucial cogs in bringing about collective change. They also, however, have their limits. Sometimes you've gotta lock arms with your fellow man, hit the streets, and exercise your First Amendment right to peacefully assemble.

IN THE WILD

Fast and easy might not be what you want to be labeled as in high school, but these tips are just that—they take just five minutes or less and are small steps that lead to big shifts over time. Try one (or many) today.

- *Request no straw or napkin when you go out for your happy hour beverage (or any beverage).*

- *Bring your own coffee cup or container to your local coffee shop today instead of relying on disposables. And if you forget your reusable, all's not lost. Carve out five minutes to enjoy that delish sip in-store in one of their mugs or glasses.*

- *When shopping this week, ask upfront for no (or an electronic) receipt, no product wrapping, and no bag.*

- *Pack your fuggin' lunch for tomorrow and, if you want to get realllllly crazy, for the rest of the week.*

- *Got hot dinner plans? Cool! Before rolling out, bring a reusable container with you so you can bring those delish leftovers home in something sturdy and less wasteful. Drunk-you will thank you tomorrow morning when you roll out of bed only to discover pristine Chana Masala well preserved in your fridge.*

- *If applicable to you, inquire about and research your company's work-from-home and charitable matching policies. Then see how that information will personally apply to you to either limit your commuting consumption or maximize your donations to sustainability-minded organizations.*

- *Need to give someone a gift? Think of secondhand or experience options. And when wrapping, use upcycled materials to preserve the magic and mystery of present-opening without adding waste to the landfill.*

- *Explore environmental, animal advocacy, and human rights organizations and political candidates in your area, and see how you can get involved.*

Conclusion

Because you've made it this far, the certifying body of Ashlee Piper, Inc. (Note: not a real company) hereby declares you ready and able to give a shit. How does it feel? Hopefully you're excited, pumped, and stoked to bust a sustainable move (or many moves). This book is a solid beginning (I may be biased), but don't let it be the end. The issues discussed herein are so complex, multifaceted, and interrelated that it's virtually impossible to thoroughly cover everything without toeing dangerously into *War and Peace* territory. And where I've left off is where you and your big beautiful brain continue the journey, well equipped and completely capable. For instance, I didn't touch on animal exploitation in working situations like horse-drawn carriages and agricultural labor, captive settings like zoos and aquariums, and entertainment industries like circuses, dog and horse racing, rodeos, bullfighting, dancing bears, and a host of other crazy shit that exists. These issues are personally important to me, and if they sound like something you wish to explore more, by golly, go forth! Limited word count and attention spans meant that I didn't cover every human rights violation, destroyed habitat, or global warming scenario in existence. You, however, should. I urge you to explore these and other issues from all perspectives and, if you're so inclined, fold them into your own value system and personal practices.

And while you're on the hunt for more knowledge and solutions, I have a hunch that some of you may be moved to transcend information gathering into tangible activism. I know this will come as a shock, but organizations advocating for the environment, exploited persons, and animals aren't exactly flush with cash. Facing down well-connected, wealthy networks of industry Goliaths requires significant fortitude, money, and manpower. When you can, give of your funds and time to organizations working tirelessly to make the world a better place. No matter the extent to which you adopt the tips in this book, most of us have some bandwidth to volunteer at a shelter or sanctuary, share legal, tech, or bookkeeping expertise with an understaffed nonprofit, or donate funds to organizations doing the challenging, scary work of dismantling entrenched networks of exploitation (I outline some of my favorite organizations at ashleepiper.com/LBB).

And you needn't wait to be legitimately indoctrinated if orientations and background checks aren't your bag. Pick up trash you see on the street or at the beach, buy a homeless person a plant-based meal, foster a senior cat, give someone struggling a job or a compliment, and, above all, lead by kind, cool, open-minded example. And if all that doesn't sate the fire in your belly, do as I did and make this passion your career. There are no limits to giving a shit. And to tie it all back to the very beginning, the beating heart of this book borrowed from Alice Walker's unfailing wisdom: *We are the ones we have been waiting for*. This means that for every problem and injustice, the solution starts with you. Singular, impassioned, informed, small-but-unbelievably-mighty you.

Acknowledgments

Writing a book is, wow, a lot of work, and I certainly didn't tackle this alone. So many people to thank, but chief among them: generous folk like Natalie Slater, Eric Lindstrom, Sally Ekus, and Heather Crosby who lent guidance when this book was just a seedling of an idea. My incredible agent, Mary, who was a believer from the beginning and provided advice, laughs, and the tenacity that kept the dream alive. The rad-as-hell Running Press team, including Frances, Seta, and especially my editor Jess, who enthusiastically rode the *Give a Sh*t* train early on and brought this book to life. Folks like Paige Vickers, Alex Zeleniuch, Adam and Kris Steele, Josephine Moore, Hope Clarke, Kendra Millis, Katie Hubbard, and Julie Ford who dotted the i's and crossed the t's to ensure this book was both beautiful and not littered with typos. Marisa for giving me my first gig in animal rights, and Andy, for believing I could do this when I didn't yet believe it myself.

Throughout, the loving encouragement from dear friends like Amber, Frank, Alisha, Amy L., Amy M., Chi, Theresa, Paley, Francine, Liz, Jessica, Chloé Jo, Kat, and Heather, just to name a few, and the support from my incredibly patient coworkers who helped me as I balanced a full-time gig whilst writing this bad boy. To my 11th grade English teacher, Mrs. Gatzlaff who, despite my truancy and terrible eyebrows, told me I "would be a writer someday" (when others said it'd be a miracle if I even got into college). Last, but certainly not least, my incomparable family who instilled early on that with hustle and heart, anything is possible: Mom, Dad, Nonna, Hattie, Mimi, Papa, Uncle Eric, Grandpa Piper, Philip, and Lavonna—you guys are my true North. And to my best pal, Banjo, and every animal I've had the honor to spend time with, without whom I'd have never written this book or understood my passion and purpose. I'm so grateful to and inspired by you all. Thank you.

Endnotes

Introduction

1 Unilever, "Report Shows a Third of Consumers Prefer Sustainable Brands," May 1, 2017, https://www.unilever.com/news/press-releases/2017/report-shows-a-third-of-consumers-prefer-sustainable-brands.html; Neilsen, "The Sustainability Imperative," October 12, 2015, www.nielsen.com/us/en/insights/reports/2015/the-sustainability-imperative.html.

2 Carbon Dioxide Information Analysis Center, 2014, http://cdiac.ess-dive.lbl.gov/trends/emis/meth_reg.html; Justin Gillis and Nadja Popovich, "The U.S. Is the Biggest Carbon Polluter in History. It Just Walked Away from the Paris Climate Deal," *New York Times*, June 1, 2017, www.nytimes.com/interactive/2017/06/01/climate/us-biggest-carbon-polluter-in-history-will-it-walk-away-from-the-paris-climate-deal.html.

3 "Climate Change: How Do We Know?"

4 Ibid.

5 "Climate Change Impacts in the United States," National Climate Assessment, http://nca2014.globalchange.gov/report/our-changing-climate/changes-hurricanes

6 Daniel Glick, "The Big Thaw," *National Geographic*, https://www.nationalgeographic.com/environment/global-warming/big-thaw/; Carol Rasmussen, "Wind, warm water revved up melting Antartctic glaciers," NASA, September 19, 2017, https://climate.nasa.gov/news/2631/wind-warm-water-revved-up-melting-antarctic-glaciers/

7 "Climate Change: How Do We Know?" NASA, https://climate.nasa.gov/evidence.

8 Michel Martin, "For the First Time in 146 Years Chicago Goes Without Snow During January and February," All Things Considered, NPR, March 4, 2017, www.npr.org/2017/03/04/518527669/for-the-first-time-in-146-years-chicago-goes-without-snow-during-january-and-feb.

9 Colin P. Kelley, Shahrzad Mohtadi, Mark A. Cane, Richard Seager, and Yochanan Kushnir, "Climate Change in the Fertile Crescent and Implications of the Recent Syrian Drought," PNAS 112, no. 11 (March 17, 2015): 3241–3246, www.pnas.org/content/112/11/3241.full.pdf; "National Security Implications of Climate-Related Risks and a Changing Climate," US Department of Defense, July 23, 2015, http://archive.defense.gov/pubs/150724-congressional-report-on-national-implications-of-climate-change.pdf?source=govdelivery.

10 Glen Althor, James E. M. Watson, and Richard A. Fuller, "Global Mismatch Between Greenhouse Gas Emissions and the Burden of Climate Change," *Scientific Reports* 6, no. 20281 (February 5, 2016), www.nature.com/articles/

srep20281.

Give a Shit: In Your Home

1 "Municipal Solid Waste," US Environmental Protection Agency, https://archive.epa.gov/epawaste/nonhaz/municipal/web/html; "Advancing Sustainable Materials Management: Facts and Figures," US Environmental Protection Agency, www.epa.gov/smm/advancing-sustainable-materials-management-facts-and-figures.

2 "Study Finds 73% of U.S. Consumers Have Access to Curbside Recycling Programs," RRS, https://recycle.com/spc-recycling-access-study.

3 Neff, Spiker, and Truant, "Wasted Food"; "Don't Waste, Donate"; QI and Roe, "Household Food Waste"; Bloom, "In United States, There's a Lot of Food Being Wasted"; "Key Statistics and Graphics," US Department of Agriculture, www.ers.usda.gov/topics/food-nutrition-assistance/food-security-in-the-us/key-statistics-graphics.aspx; "Food Waste," Grace Communications Foundation, www.sustainabletable.org/5664/food-waste.

4 Sustainable Management of Food Basics," US Environmental Protection Agency, www.epa.gov/sustainable-management-food/sustainable-management-food-basics.

5 Elizabeth Brackett, "Where Does Chicago's Trash Go?" WTTW, June 26, 2017, http://chicagotonight.wttw.com/2017/06/26/where-does-chicagos-garbage-go.

6 Alana Semuels, "Charging for Trash, Bag by Bag," *Atlantic*, August 18, 2015, www.theatlantic.com/business/archive/2015/08/charging-for-trash-bag-by-bag/425907.

7 Viviana Solorzano and Andrew Edwards, "Memo: Executive Summary Report—Composting," Harris Interactive, December 27, 2013, www.recycle.cc/2013-1227NW&RA_composting_survey_executive_summary_010814.pdf. "How Much Energy Is Consumed in U.S. Residential and Commercial Buildings?"; "Consumption and Efficiency"; Tariq Khokhar, "Chart: Over 1 Billion People Had No Access to Electricity in 2014," The Data Blog, World Bank, April 3, 2017, https://blogs.worldbank.org/opendata/chartover-1-billion-people-had-no-access-electricity-2014; Nargi, "Think Your Household Is Sustainable? Think Again."

8 "Use Power Strips to Avoid Phantom Loads," Wisconsin Public Service, https://accel.wisconsinpublicservice.com/home/tips/electronics_powerstrips.aspx; Brian Palmer, "Keep Your Devices from Wasting Energy and Money," Natural Resources Defense Council, December 31, 2015, www.nrdc.org/stories/keep-your-devices-wasting-energy-and-money.

9 Palmer, "Keep Your Devices from Wasting Energy and Money"; Michael Casey, "Always-On Devices Are Using Huge Amounts of Energy," *CBS News*, May 8, 2015, www.cbsnews.com/news/always-on-devices-are-using-huge-amounts-of-energy.

10 Selene Aparicio, "Shut the Fridge Door—You're Wasting Electricity," *Good Housekeeping*, February 8, 2014, www.goodhousekeeping.com/home/a19095/refrigerator-door-wastes-energy.

11 "How Much Energy Is Used for Lighting in the United States?" Frequently Asked Questions, U.S. Energy Information Administration, www.eia.gov/tools/faqs/faq.php?id=99&t=3.

12 "Lower Your Light Bill and Save Energy," *Good Housekeeping*, February 21, 2008.

13 "How Energy-Efficient Light Bulbs Compare with Traditional Incandescents," Energy.gov, https://energy.gov/energysaver/how-energy-efficient-light-bulbs-compare-traditional-incandescents.

14 Ibid.

15 "Showerheads," US Environmental Protection Agency, www.epa.gov/sites/production/files/2017-01/documents/ws-products-factsheet-showerheads.pdf; Debbie Arrington, "Showers vs. Baths: Which Use Less Water?" *Sacramento Bee*, February 13, 2014, www.sacbee.com/news/state/california/water-and-drought/article2591077.html; "How to Save Water," Water Footprint Calculator, www.watercalculator.org/save-water/?cid=437.

16 Ibid.

17 "Bathroom Faucets," U.S. Environmental Protection Agency, www.epa.gov/watersense/bathroom-faucets.

18 "Residential Toilets," U.S. Environmental Protection Agency, www.epa.gov/watersense/residential-toilets.

19 "5 No-Nonsense Ways to Cut Your Water Heater Energy Costs," House Logic, www.houselogic.com/organize-maintain/home-maintenance-tips/water-heater-energy-saving-tips.

20 Ibid.

21 "Watering Tips," US Environmental Protection Agency, www.epa.gov/watersense/watering-tips.

22 "How Is Electricity Used in U.S. Homes?" Frequently Asked Questions, US Energy Information Administration, www.eia.gov/tools/faqs/faq.php?id=96&t=3.

23 "How to Cool a Hot Attic," HGTV, www.hgtv.com/design/decorating/clean-and-organize/how-to-cool-a-hot-attic.

24 "Whole House Fan," US Department of Energy, www.nrel.gov/docs/fy99osti/26291.pdf.

25 B. C. Wolverton, Willard L. Douglas, and Keith Bounds, "A Study of Interior Landscape Plants for Indoor Air Pollution Abatement," NASA, July 1, 1989, https://ntrs.nasa.gov/search.jsp?R=19930072988.

26 "Indoor Air Quality," EPA's Report on the Environment, US Environmental Protection Agency, https://cfpub.epa.gov/roe/chapter/air/indoorair.cfm.

27 Wolverton, Douglas, and Bounds, "A Study of Interior Landscape Plants for Indoor Air Pollution Abatement."

28 MacVean, "For Many People, Gathering Possessions Is Just the Stuff of Life."

29 "Clean Freaks" *Newsweek*, June 6, 2004, www.newsweek.com/clean-freaks-129009.

30 Miranda Bryant, "The REAL Cost of Keeping Your Home Tidy: Americans Spend $140,000 in Their Lifetimes and 30 Days Every Year on Boring Household Tasks Like Cleaning and Laundry," *Daily Mail*, March 28, 2016, www.dailymail.co.uk/femail/article-3512386/The-REAL-cost-keeping-home-tidy-Americans-spend-140-000-lifetimes-30-days-year-boring-household-tasks-like-cleaning-laundry.html; "Charts by Topic: Household Activities," American Time Use Survey, US Bureau of Labor Statistics, www.bls.gov/TUS/CHARTS/HOUSEHOLD.HTM.

31 "You can also define things that spark joy as things that make you happy." Marie Kondo, *Spark Joy: An Illustrated Master Class on the Art of Organizing and Tidying Up* (Berkeley, CA: Ten Speed Press, 2016), 82.

32 "Junk Mail Facts," US Junk Mail, www.usjunkmail.com/consumer/factsOther.aspx.

33 "Junk Mail," NYU Law, www.law.nyu.edu/about/sustainability/whatyoucando/junkmail.

34 "Is 7 Your Lucky Number?" Knowledge Marketing, www.knowledgemarketing.com/index.php/7-lucky-number.

35 "Stopping Unsolicited Mail, Phone Calls, and Email," Consumer Information, Federal Trade Commission, www.consumer.ftc.gov/articles/0262-stopping-unsolicited-mail-phone-calls-and-email.

36 Ann Carrns, "Before Giving, Check Out Charities and Their Policies on Privacy," *New York Times*, December 1, 2015, www.nytimes.com/2015/12/02/your-money/before-giving-check-out-charities-and-their-policies-on-privacy.html.

37 "EPA Reports 9.8 Million Tons Per Year in Furniture Waste," Reuters, May 6, 2011, www.reuters.com/article/idUS126369713020110506.

38 "Planned Obsolescence," Wikipedia, https://en.wikipedia.org/wiki/Planned_obsolescence.

39 Lore Leibovich, "Turn Off the Tube, Have More Sex," *Salon*, January 17, 2006, www.salon.com/2006/01/17/sex_tv.

40 Andrew Van Dam and Eric Morath, "Changing Times: How Americans Spend Their Day Reflects a Shifting Economy and Population," *Wall Street Journal*, June 24, 2016, https://graphics.wsj.com/time-use.

41 Claire Landsbaum, "How Gross Is Your Mattress?" *Slate*, November 24, 2105, www.slate.com/blogs/the_drift/2015/1½4/mattresses_dust_mites_and_skin_cells_how_gross_does_your_mattress_get_over.html.

42 Gary James, "Mattress Certifications, Standards, Seals, Tags and Labels," *BedTimes*, November 2012, https://bedtimesmagazine.com/2012/11/certifications-standards-seals-tags-labels-key-programs-for-the-u-s-bedding-industry.

43 "Use Power Strips to Avoid Phantom Loads"; Palmer, "Keep Your Devices from Wasting Energy and Money."

44 Dan Stone, "Laptop vs. PC Power Consumption," Chron, http://smallbusiness.chron.com/laptop-vs-pc-power-consumption-79347.html.

45 "American Time Use Survey Summary," Economic New Release," US Bureau of Labor Statistics, June 27, 2017, www.bls.gov/news.release/atus.nr0.htm.

46 "Electricity Usage of a Clothes Washer," EnergyUse Calculator, http://energyusecalculator.com/electricity_clotheswasher.htm.

47 "'Greener' Laundry by the Load: Fabric Softener versus Dryer Sheets," *Scientific American*, www.scientificamerican.com/article/greener-laundry.

48 Mandi Woodruff, "Your Dry Cleaning Bill Is About to Get Even More Expensive," *Business Insider*, June 4, 2012, www.businessinsider.com/get-ready-to-pay-more-for-your-dry-cleaning-bill-2012-6.

49 "Clothes Washers," Certified Products, Energy Star, www.energystar.gov/products/appliances/clothes_washers.

50 Mark Bittman, "A No-Frills Kitchen Still Cooks," *New York Times*, May 9, 2007, www.nytimes.com/2007/05/09/dining/09mini.html.

51 Marie Doezema, "Consumers Are Dumping Keurig's Single-Serve Coffee—And That's Great News for the Environment," *Vice*, February 13, 2016, https://news.vice.com/article/consumers-are-dumping-keurigs-single-serve-coffee-and-thats-great-news-for-the-environment.

52 "Cleaning Supplies and Your Health," Environmental Working Group, www.ewg.org/guides/cleaners/content/cleaners_and_health#.WgR96UxFzXd; "Worst Cleaners: EWG's List of Most Harmful Cleaning Products for Your Home," *Huffington Post*, September 10, 2012, www.huffingtonpost.com/2012/09/10/worst-household-cleaners-cleaning-products_n_1871420.html.

Give a Shit: In the Kitchen

1 Food and Agricultural Organization of the United Nations, "Livestock's Long Shadow: Environmental Issues and Options," United Nations, Rome, 2006, www.fao.org/docrep/010/a0701e/a0701e00.HTM.

2 "Meat Consumption," Data, OECD, https://data.oecd.org/agroutput/meat-consumption.htm.

3 "Livestock and Climate Change: What If the Key Actors in Climate Change Are Cows, Pigs, and Chickens?" World Watch, November–December 2009, www.worldwatch.org/files/pdf/Livestock%20and%20Climate%20Change.pdf; Food and Agricultural Organization of the United Nations, "Livestock's Long Shadow"; Food and Agricultural Organization of the United Nations, "Tackling Climate Change Through Livestock—A Global Assessment of Emissions and Mitigation Opportunities," www.fao.org/3/a-i3437e/index.html.

4 "A Closer Look at Animals on Factory Farms," Farm Animal Welfare, ASPCA, www.aspca.org/animal-cruelty/farm-animal-welfare/animals-factory-farms; "Why Are CAFOs Bad?" Michigan Chapter, Sierra Club, www.sierraclub.org/michigan/why-are-cafos-bad; "At a Glance," US Environmental Protection Agency, Office of Inspector General, September 19, 2017, www.epa.gov/sites/production/files/2017-09/documents/_epaoig_20170919-17-p-0396_glance.pdf; "Ending Factory Farming," Farm Forward, https://farmforward.com/ending-factory-farming (Farm Forward calculation based on US Department of Agriculture, 2012 Census of Agriculture, June 2014).

5 Food and Agricultural Organization of the United Nations, "Tackling Climate Change Through Livestock"; "Cattle," USDA, July 21, 2017, http://usda.mannlib.cornell.edu/usda/current/Catt/Catt-07-21-2017.pdf.

6 "Waste Management," Grace Communications Foundation, www.sustainabletable.org/906/waste-management.

7 Gowri Koneswaran and Danielle Nierenberg, "Global Farm Animal Productions and Global Warming: Impacting and Mitigating Climate Change," Environmental Health Perspectives 116, no. 5 (May 2008), www.ncbi.nlm.nih.gov/pmc/articles/PMC2367646.

8 "Concentrated Animal Feeding Operation," Wikipedia, https://en.wikipedia.org/wiki/Concentrated_animal_feeding_operation.

9 "Animal Manure Management," USDA, RCA Issue Brief #7, December 1995, www.nrcs.usda.gov/wps/portal/nrcs/detail/null/?cid=nrcs143_014211; "Agricultural Waste Management Field Handbook," USDA, https://directives.sc.egov.usda.gov/viewerFS.aspx?hid=21430.

10 "Pollution (Water, Air, Chemicals)," Food Empowerment Project, www.foodispower.org/pollution-water-air-chemicals; "Waste Management," Grace Communications Foundation.

11 "Risk Assessment Evaluation for Concentrated Animal Feeding Operations," US Environmental Protection Agency, http://bit.ly/2mh06ST.

12 "Industrial Farm Animal Production," National Commission on Industrial Farm Animal Production, www.ncifap.org/reports.

13 Chad Heeter, "The Oil in Your Oatmeal: A Lot of Fossil Fuel Goes into Producing, Packaging and Shipping Our Breakfast," San Francisco Gate, March 26, 2006, www.sfgate.com/opinion/article/The-oil-in-your-oatmeal-A-lot-of-fossil-fuel-2501200.php.

14 R. L. Huffman and P. W. Westerman, "Estimated Seepage Losses from Established Swine Waste Lagoons in the Lower Coastal Plain in North Carolina," *Transactions of the American Society of Agricultural Engineers* 38, no. 2 (1995): 449–453; Environmental Protection Agency, "National Pollutant Discharge Elimination System Permit Regulation and Effluent Limitation Guidelines and Standards for Concentrated Animal Feeding Operations; Proposed Rule," Federal Register, January 12, 2001, www.gpo.gov/fdsys/pkg/FR-2001-01-12/pdf/01-1.pdf.

15 Marcel P. Aillery, Neol R. Gollehon, Robert C. Johansson, Jonathan D. Kaplan, and Nigel D. Key, "Managing Manure to Improve Air and Water Quality," *USDA Economic Research Report* 9 (January 1, 2005).

16 Farm Safety Association, "Manure Gas Dangers," 2002, www.nasdonline.org/static_content/documents/48/d001616.pdf.

17 Andrew D. McEachran, Brett R. Blackwell, J. Delton Hanson, Kimberly J. Wooten, Gregory D. Mayer, Stephen B. Cox, and Philip N. Smith, "Antibiotics, Bacteria, and Antibiotic Resistance Genes: Aerial Transport from Cattle Feed Yards via Particulate Matter," Environmental Health Perspectives, January 22, 2015, https://ehp.niehs.nih.gov/wp-content/uploads/advpub/2015/1/ehp.1408555.acco.pdf; Tom Philpott, "Dust from Factory Farms Carries Drugs, Poop Bacteria, and Antibiotic-Resistant Genes Far and Wide," *Mother Jones*, January 27, 2015, www.motherjones.com/food/2015/01/dust-factory-farms-antibiotic-resistant-genes.

18 UN Conference on Trade and Development, "Wake Up Before It Is Too Late," Trade and Environment Review, 2013, http://unctad.org/en/PublicationsLibrary/ditcted2012d3_en.pdf; "Livestock a Major Threat to Environment," FAO Newsroom, November 29, 2006, www.fao.org/newsroom/en/News/2006/1000448/index.html; Bryan Walsh, "The Triple Whopper Environmental Impact of Global Meat Production," *TIME*, December 16, 2013, science.time.com/2013/12/16/the-triple-whopper-environmental-impact-of-global-meat-production; Phillip Thornton, Mario Herrero, and Polly Ericksen, "Livestock and Climate Change," *Livestock xchange*, November 2011, https://cgspace.cgiar.org/bitstream/handle/10568/10601/IssueBrief3.pdf; Pete Smith and Mercedes Bustamante et al., "Agriculture, Forestry and Other Land Use (AFOLU)," Intergovernmental Panel on Climate Change, chapter 11, www.ipcc.ch/pdf/assessment-report/ar5/wg3/ipcc_wg3_ar5_chapter11.pdf

19 "Farms and Farmland," USDA Census of Agriculture, September 2014, https://www.agcensus.usda.gov/Publications/2012/Online_Resources/Highlights/Farms_and_Farmland/Highlights_Farms_and_Farmland.pdf.

20 Sergio Margulis, "Causes of Deforestation of the Brazilian Amazon." World Bank Working Paper no. 22., 2003, http://documents.worldbank.org/curated/en/758171468768828889/pdf/277150PAPER0wbwp0no1022.pdf; Hiroko Tabuchi, Claire Rigby, and Jeremy White, "Amazon Deforestation, Once TameD, Comes Roaring Back," *New York Times*, February 24, 2017, www.nytimes.com/2017/02/24/business/energy-environment/deforestation-brazil-bolivia-south-america.html?_r=0; Marisa Bellantonio, Glenn Hurowitz, Anne Leifsdatter Grønlund, and Anahita Yousefi, "The Ultimate Mystery Meat: Exposing the Secrets Behind Burger King and Global Meat Production," Mighty Earth, www.mightyearth.org/mysterymeat; Richard A. Oppenlander, *Food Choice and Sustainability: Why Buying Local, Eating Less Meat, and Taking Baby Steps Won't Work* (Minneapolis, MN: Langdon Street Press, 2013).

21 "Measuring the Daily Destruction of the World's Rainforests." *Scientific American*, www.scientificamerican.com/article/earth-talks-daily-destruction; Rhett Butler, "10 Rainforest Facts for 2017," Mongabay, January 2, 2017, https://rainforests.mongabay.com/facts/rainforest-facts.html#8; "Tropical Deforestation," NASA Facts, November 1998, https://msu.edu/~urquhart/professional/NASA-Deforestation.pdf.

22 John Vidal, "Protect Nature for World Economic Security, Warns UN Biodiversity Chief," *Guardian*, August 16, 2010, www.theguardian.com/environment/2010/aug/16/nature-economic-security.

23 https://phys.org/news/2017-02-carbon-uptake-amazon-forests-region.html

24 Shasta Darlington, "'Uncontacted' Amazon Tribe Members Reported Killed in Brazil," *New York Times*, September 10, 2017, www.nytimes.com/2017/09/10/world/americas/brazil-amazon-tribe-killings.html; "The Uncontacted Indians of Brazil," Survival International, www.survivalinternational.org/tribes/uncontacted-brazil.

25 "What Is Acid Rain?" US Environmental Protection Agency, www.epa.gov/acidrain/what-acid-rain.

26 "Program Data Report Part G—2016: Animals Dispersed / Killed or Euthanized / Removed or Destroyed / Freed," USDA, Animal and Plant Health Inspection Service, www.aphis.usda.gov/wildlife_damage/pdr/PDR-G_Report.php?fy=2016&fld=&fld_val=.

27 "Memo," Bureau Land Management, www.blm.gov/basic/programs-wild-horse-and-burro-news-fy18-budget-statement; Karin Brulliard and Juliet Eilperin, "Wild Horses Could Be Sold for Slaughter or Euthanized Under Trump Budget," *Washington Post*, May 26, 2017, www.washingtonpost.com/news/animalia/wp/2017/05/26/wild-horses-could-be-sold-for-slaughter-or-euthanized-under-trump-budget/?utm_term=.93a65bde6cac; "Reality of Wild Horse Slaughter," Wild Horse Education, https://wildhorseeducation.org/reality-of-wild-horse-slaughter.

28 Rae Price, "Wild Horse Advisory Board Makes Recommendations," *Western Livestock Journal*, November 1, 2017, www.wlj.net/top_headlines/wild-horse-advisory-board-makes-recommendations/article_722b9b04-bf47-11e7-bca8-dfa195def08b.html; Scott Sonner, "Trump Budget Would Allow Sale of Wild Horses for Slaughter," *Denver Post*, May 25, 2107, www.denverpost.com/2017/05/25/trump-budget-wild-horses-slaughter; "Press Release: Cattlemen, Western Ranchers Applaud Adoption of Wild Horse and Burro Management Amendment," National Cattlemen's Beef Association, www.

beefusa.org/newsreleases1.aspx?NewsID=6366.

29 Mesfin M. Mekonnen and Arjen Y. Hoekstra, "A Global Assessment of the Water Footprint of Farm Animal Products," *Ecosystems* 15 (2012): 401–415, http://temp.waterfootprint.org/Reports/Mekonnen-Hoekstra-2012-WaterFootprintFarmAnimalProducts.pdf; P. W. Gerbens-Leenes, M. M. Mekonnen, and A. Y. Hoekstra, "The Water Footprint of Poultry, Pork and Beef: A Comparative Study in Different Countries and Production Systems," *Water Resources and Industry* 1–2 (March–June 2013), 25–36; Mario Herrero, Petr Havlik, Hugo Valin, An Notenbaert, Mariana C. Rufino, Philip K. Thornton, Michael Blümmel et al., "Biomass Use, Production, Feed Efficiencies, and Greenhouse Gas Emissions from Global Livestock Systems," *Proceedings of the National Academy of Sciences* 110 no. 52 (2013), www.pnas.org/content/110/52/20888.full; Richard Oppenlander. "Freshwater Abuse and Loss: Where Is It All Going?" Forks Over Knives, May 20, 2013, www.forksoverknives.com/freshwater-abuse-and-loss-where-is-it-all-going/#gs.adhr4yw; "Drinking-Water," World Health Organization, www.who.int/mediacentre/factsheets/fs391/en.

30 "The Facts," Cowspiracy, www.cowspiracy.com/facts; Barb Glen, "Do the Math for Proper Pasture Populations," The Western Producer, February 9, 2012, www.producer.com/2012/02/do-the-math-for-proper-pasture-populations.

31 "Agriculture, Energy, & Climate Change," Grace Communications Foundation, www.sustainabletable.org/982/agriculture-energy-climate-change.

32 Jess McNally, "Can Vegetarianism Save the World? Nitty-Gritty," Stanford Alumni, https://alumni.stanford.edu/get/page/magazine/article/?article_id=29892; Lucas Reijnders and Sam Soret, "Quantification of the Environmental Impact of Different Dietary Protein Choices," *American Journal of Clinical Nutrition* 78, no. 3 (September 2003): 6645–6685, http://ajcn.nutrition.org/content/78/3/664S.full.

33 Peter Walker, "Yemen Civil War: Widespread Starvation Forces People to Eat Food from Rubbish Dumps," *Independent*, January 9, 2017, www.independent.co.uk/news/world/middle-east/yemen-civil-war-latest-starvation-eating-rubbish-dumps-sanaa-children-a7516796.html.

34 Food and Agriculture Organization of the United Nations, "How Close Are We to #ZeroHunger?" United Nations, www.fao.org/state-of-food-security-nutrition/en.

35 Eric Holt-Giménez, Annie Shattuck, Miguel Altieri, Hans Herren and Steve Gliessman, "We Already Grow Enough Food for 10 Billion People . . . and Still Can't End Hunger," *Journal of Sustainable Agriculture* 36, no. 6 (2012): 595–598, www.tandfonline.com/doi/abs/10.1080/10440046.2012.695331.

36 "The Facts," Cowspiracy; Richard Oppenlander, "The World Hunger-Food Choice Connection: A Summary," Comfortably Unaware Blog, August 2012,

comfortablyunaware.com/blog/the-world-hunger-food-choice-connection-a-summary; "Improving Child Nutrition: The Achievable Imperative for Global Progress," UNICEF, April 2013, www.unicef.org/gambia/Improving_Child_Nutrition_-_the_achievable_imperative_for_global_progress.pdf; Livestock Production Index," World Bank, https://data.worldbank.org/indicator/AG.PRD.LVSK.XD; Global Livestock Production Systems," Food and Agriculture Organization of the United Nations, Rome, 2011, www.fao.org/docrep/014/i2414e/i2414e.pdf.

37 Paul Solotaroff, "In the Belly of the Beast," *Rolling Stone*, December 10, 2013, www.rollingstone.com/feature/belly-beast-meat-factory-farms-animal-activists; "Overview of the United States Slaughter Industry," USDA, October 27, 2016, http://usda.mannlib.cornell.edu/usda/current/SlauOverview/SlauOverview-10-27-2016.pdf; Bartholomew D. Sullivan, "Congressional Panel Permits Culling of Wild Horses," *USA Today*, July 19, 2017, www.usatoday.com/story/news/politics/2017/07/19/culling-wcongressional-panel-permits-culling-wild-horses/492056001.

38 United States Code Annotated, Title 7, Agriculture, Chapter 48, Humane Methods of Livestock Slaughter, Michigan State Animal Law Center, www.animallaw.info/statute/us-food-animal-humane-methods-livestock-slaughter.

39 "Vegan 101: Your Easy Introduction to Going Vegan," PETA, https://www.peta.org/living/food/vegan-101-guide-for-new-vegans.

40 "Humane Slaughter?" Humane Facts, humanefacts.org/humane-slaughter.

41 "Humane Slaughter?"; "Cruel Slaughter Practices," Humane Society of the United States, www.humanesociety.org/issues/slaughter/?credit=mr_st_pe; "Overview of the US Slaughter Industry," USDA; Title 9, USDA, Michigan State University Animal Legal and Historical Center, www.animallaw.info/administrative/us-slaughter-humane-slaughter-livestock-regulations; "Cow Transport and Slaughter," PETA, www.peta.org/issues/animals-used-for-food/factory-farming/cows/cow-transport-slaughter; "Processing: How Are Chickens Slaughtered and Processed for Meat?" Chicken Check In, www.chickencheck.in/faq/how-chickens-slaughtered-processed; "National Chicken Council Brief on Stunning of Chickens," National Chicken Council, February 8, 2013, www.nationalchickencouncil.org/national-chicken-council-brief-on-stunning-of-chickens; Kimberly Kindy, "USDA Plan to Speed Up Poultry-Processing Lines Could Increase Risk of Bird Abuse," *Washington Post*, October 29, 2013, www.washingtonpost.com/politics/usda-plan-to-speed-up-poultry-processing-lines-could-increase-risk-of-bird-abuse/2013/10/29/aeeffe1e-3b2e-11e3-b6a9-da62c264f40e_story.html?utm_term=.b2053381b4ad; Nico Pitney, "Scientists Believe the Chickens We Eat Are Being Slaughtered While Conscious," *Huffington Post*, October 28, 2016, www.huffingtonpost.com/entry/chickens-slaughtered-conscious_us_580e3d3e4b000d0b157bf98; Charlotte Berg and Mohan Raj, "A Review of Stunning Methods for Poultry—Animal Welfare Aspects," *Animals* 5, no. 4 (December 2015): 1207–1219), /www.ncbi.nlm.nih.gov/pmc/articles/

PMC4693211; "Regulatory Definitions of Large CAFOs, Mediums CAFO, and CAFOs," US Environmental Protection Agency, www3.epa.gov/npdes/pubs/sector_table.pdf; David Montgomery, "Washington Post Profiles COK! Animal Pragmatism: Compassion Over Killing Wants to Make the Anti Meat Message a Little More Palatable," Web Citation, September 8, 2003, https://www.webcitation.org/6DIAXlvM8?url=http://www.cok.net/feat/article-wp.php. Venessa Wong, "Egg Makers Are Freaked Out by the Cage-Free Future," CNBC, March 22, 2017, https://www.cnbc.com/2017/03/22/egg-makers-are-freaked-out-by-the-cage-free-future.html. "Cage-Free vs. Battery-Cage Eggs: Comparison of Animal Welfare in Both Methods," The Humane Society of the United States, http://www.humanesociety.org/issues/confinement_farm/facts/cage-free_vs_battery-cage.html?credit=blog_post2415. "Scientists and Experts on Battery Cages and Laying Hen Welfare," The Humane Society of the United States, http://www.humanesociety.org/assets/pdfs/farm/HSUS-Synopsis-of-Expert-Opinions-on-Battery-Cages-and-Hen-Welfare.pdf. "Animal Husbandry Guidelines for U.S. Egg Laying Flocks: 2016 Edition," United Egg Producers Certified, https://uepcertified.com/wp-content/uploads/2015/08/2016-UEP-Animal-Welfare-Guidelines-2016-Cage-Free-Edit-002.pdf "Rules and Regulations," Federal Register, Vol. 81, No. 137, July 18, 2016, https://www.fsis.usda.gov/wps/wcm/connect/3e42d239-982d-4634-9b51-d7189a08ce71/2014-0020.pdf?MOD=AJPERES. "Compliance Guidelines for Use of Video or Other Electronic Monitoring or Recording Equipment in Federally Inspected Establishments," United States Department of Agriculture Food Safety and Inspection Service, https://www.fsis.usda.gov/wps/wcm/connect/5905b82f-3579-4e0f-beb2-5b860cc0b087/Compliance_Guidelines_for_Use_of_Video_082611.pdf?MOD=AJPERES. "Inhumane Handling of Livestock in Connection With Slaughter by Persons Not Employed by the Official Establishment," Federal Register, October 26, 2016, https://www.federalregister.gov/documents/2016/10/26/2016-24754/inhumane-handling-of-livestock-in-connection-with-slaughter-by-persons-not-employed-by-the-official. "Humane Handling and Slaughter of Livestock," United States Department of Agriculture Food Safety and Inspection Service, August 15, 2011, https://www.fsis.usda.gov/wps/wcm/connect/2375f4d5-0e24-4213-902d-d94ee4ed9394/6900.2.pdf?MOD=AJPERES. "Regulatory Compliance: Humane Handling," United States Department of Agriculture Food Safety and Inspection Service, https://www.fsis.usda.gov/wps/portal/fsis/topics/regulatory-compliance/humane-handling. "United States Code Annotated, Title 49, Transportation, Subtitle X, Miscellaneous, Chapter 805, Miscellaneous," Michigan State Animal Law Center, July, 2016, https://www.animallaw.info/statute/us-food-animal-twenty-eight-hour-law. "Perspective on Transportation Issues: The Importance of Having Physically Fit Cattle and Pigs," Colorado State University Department of Animal Sciences, July 2000, http://www.grandin.com/behaviour/perspectives.transportation.issues.html. "Reproduction Practices on U.S. Dairy Operations, 2007," United States Department of Agriculture Animal and Plant Health Inspection Service, February 2009, https://www.aphis.usda.gov/animal_health/nahms/dairy/

downloads/dairy07/Dairy07_is_ReprodPrac.pdf. "Food Safety Information: Veal from Farm to Table," United States Department of Agriculture Food Safety and Inspection Service, https://www.fsis.usda.gov/wps/wcm/connect/c1c3ed6a-c1e5-4ad0-ba6c-d53d71d741c6/Veal_from_Farm_to_Table.pdf?MOD=AJPERES. "Questions," American Veal Association, http://www.americanveal.com/questions/. "Organic Livestock and Poultry Practices Final Rule," United States Department of Agriculture Agricultural Marking Service, January 2017, https://www.ams.usda.gov/sites/default/files/media/OLPPExternalQA.pdf.

42 Southern Poverty Law Center, USDA lawsuit, September 3, 2013, www.fsis.usda.gov/wps/wcm/connect/cab74978-9bac-4768-ad23-c11ff91e7257/Petition-Southern-Poverty-Law-Center-090313.pdf?MOD=AJPERES; "Slaughterhouse Workers," Food Empowerment Project, www.foodispower.org/slaughterhouse-workers; William Kandel, "Recent Trends in Rural-Based Meat Processing," Economic Research Service, presented at Immigration Reform: Implications for Farmers, Farm Workers, and Communities Conference, Washington, DC, May 21–22, 2009, https://migrationfiles.ucdavis.edu/uploads/cf/files/2009-may/kandel.pdf; Human Rights Watch, "Blood, Sweat and Fear: Workers' Rights in U.S. Meat and Poultry Plants," 2004, www.hrw.org/reports/2005/usa0105; F. William Engdahl, "Bird Flu and Chicken Factory Farms: Profit Bonanza for US Agribusiness," Global Research, November 27, 2005, www.engdahl.oilgeopolitics.net/print/Bird%20Flu%20and%20Chicken%20Factory%20Farms.htm.

43 Anna Dorovskikh, "Killing for a Living: Psychological and Physiological Effects of Alienation of Food Production on Slaughterhouse Workers," Undergraduate Honors Thesis, University of Colorado, Boulder, Spring 2015, https://scholar.colorado.edu/honr_theses/771; A. J. Fitzgerald, "A Social History of the Slaughterhouse: From Inception to Contemporary Implications," *Human Ecology Review* 17, no. 1 (2010), 58–69.

44 E. Cudworth, "Climate Change, Industrial Animal Agriculture and Complex Inequalities," *International Journal of Science in Society* 2, no. 3 (2011): 323–335; Dorovskikh, "Killing for a Living"; Eric Schlosser, "How to Make the Country's Most Dangerous Job Safer," *Atlantic*, January 2002, www.theatlantic.com/magazine/archive/2002/01/how-to-make-the-countrys-most-dangerous-job-safer/302395; "New Release: Nonfatal Occupational Injuries and Illnesses Requiring Days Away from Work," U.S. Bureau of Labor Statistics, November 10, 2016, www.bls.gov/news.release/pdf/osh2.pdf.

45 Rachel M. MacNair, *Perpetration-Induced Traumatic Stress: The Psychological Consequences of Killing* (New York: Authors Choice Press, 2005); Jennifer Dillard, "A Slaughterhouse Nightmare: Psychological Harm Suffered by Slaughterhouse Employees and the Possibility of Redress Through Legal Reform," *Georgetown Journal on Poverty Law & Policy*, 15, no. 2 (2008): 391–408; Grant Gerlock, "We Don't Know How Many Workers Are Injured at Slaughterhouse. Here's Why," NPR, May 25, 2016, https://www.npr.org/sections/thesalt/2016/05/25/479509221/we-dont-know-how-many-workers-are-injured-at-slaughterhouses-heres-why. "Workplace Safety and Health: Safety in the Meat and Poultry Industry, While Improving, Could Be Further Strengthened", U.S. Government Accountability Office, January 12, 2005, https://www.gao.gov/products/GAO-05-96. Jessica G. Ramsey, et al., "Evaluation of Carpal Tunnel Syndrom and Other Musculoskeletal Disorders among Employees at a Poultry Processing Plant," Center for Disease Control, June 2015, https://www.cdc.gov/niosh/hhe/reports/pdfs/2014-0040-3232. pdf. "No Relief: Denial of Bathroom Breaks in the Poultry Industry," OXFAM America, May 9, 2016, https://www.oxfamamerica.org/explore/research-publications/no-relief/. Peggy Lowe, "Working 'The Chain,' Slaughterhouse Workers Face Lifelong Injuries", NPR August 11, 2016, https://www.npr.org/sections/thesalt/2016/08/11/489468205/working-the-chain-slaughterhouse-workers-face-lifelong-injuries. Peggy Lowe, "Dangerous Jobs, Cheap Meat: Working 'The Chain,' Slaughterhouse Workers Face Lifelong Injuries," Flatland, June 15, 2016, http://www.flatlandkc.org/news-issues/special-reports/dangerous-jobs-cheap-meat-working-the-chain-slaughterhouse-workers-face-life-long-injuries/. "Workplace Safety and Health: Better Outreach, Collaboration, and Information Needed to Help Protect Workers at Meat and Poultry Plants," U.S. Government Accountability Office, December 7, 2017, https://www.gao.gov/products/GAO-18-12?utm_medium=email&utm_source=govdelivery. Anna Casey, "From Amputations to Respiratory Illness, New Report Exposes Hazards of Slaughterhouse Work," December 15, 2017, http://inthesetimes.com/working/entry/20771/meat-processing-slaughterhouse-workers-government-accountability-office.

46 Gail Eisnitz, *Slaughterhouse: The Shocking Story of Greed, Neglect, and Inhumane Treatment Inside the U.S. Meat Industry* (Amherst, NY: Prometheus Books, 2007); James McWilliams, "PTSD in the Slaughterhouse," *Texas Observer*, February 7, 2012; Dillard, "A Slaughterhouse Nightmare."

47 Amy J. Fitzgerald, Linda Kalof, and Thomas Dietz, "Slaughterhouses and Increased Crime Rates: An Empirical Analysis of the Spillover from 'The Jungle' into the Surrounding Community," *Organization & Environment* 22, no. 2 (June 2009): 158–184.

48 Eisnitz, *Slaughterhouse*, 57.

49 Dillard, " A Slaughterhouse Nightmare."

50 Kristen Fischer, "Why Vegetarians Are Thinner Than You," *Prevention*, November 18, 2013, www.prevention.com/food/healthy-eating-tips/vegetarian-diet-linked-sustained-weight-loss; Vesanto Melina, Winston, Craig, and Susan Levin, "Position of the Academy of Nutrition and Dietetics: Vegetarian Diets," *Journal of the Academy of Nutrition and Dietetics* 116, no. 12 (December 2016): 1970–1980.

51 Michael Nedelman, "Should You Take Statins? Two Guidelines Offer Different Answers," CNN Health, April 18, 2017, www.cnn.com/2017/04/18/health/statins-guidelines-conflict-study/index.html; Brady Dennis, "Nearly 60 Percent of Americans—the Highest Ever—Are Taking Prescription Drugs,"

Washington Post, November 3, 2015, www.washingtonpost.com/news/to-your-health/wp/2015/11/03/more-americans-than-ever-are-taking-prescription-drugs/?utm_term=.0eccabfef895.

52 Laura McMullen, "7 Reason to Choos a Plant-Based Diet," *US News and World Report*, January 5, 2016, https://health.usnews.com/health-news/health-wellness/slideshows/reasons-to-choose-a-plant-based-diet; "Plant-Based Diets," NutritionFacts.org, https://nutritionfacts.org/topics/plant-based-diets; Lizette Borreli, "Go Vegan for Your Sex Drive: 6 Reasons Veganism Holds the Key for a Healthy Sex Life," Medical Daily, April 7, 2014, www.medicaldaily.com/go-vegan-your-sex-drive-6-reasons-veganism-holds-key-healthy-sex-life-275068; Madeline Haller, "The Sex Secret Vegans Know," *Men's Health*, November 13, 2012, www.menshealth.com/sex-women/the-sex-secret-vegans-know.

53 "Chapter 6: Transport of Livestock," FAO, www.fao.org/docrep/003/x6909e/x6909e08.htm.

54 Sy Montgomery, "Giant Pacific Octopus: The Alien at Your Doorstep," *Seattle Times*, May 29, 2015, www.seattletimes.com/opinion/giant-pacific-octopus-the-alien-at-your-doorstep.

55 Iben Meyer and Björn Forkman, "Nonverbal Communication and Human-Dog Interaction," *Anthrozoös* 27, no. 4, (2014): 553–568.

56 Frans de Waal, *Are We Smart Enough to Know How Smart Animals Are?* (London: Granta Books, 2017).

57 Adam Boult, "Crows Are Surprisingly Good at Making Tools, Study Finds," *Telegraph*, August 10, 2016, www.telegraph.co.uk/news/2016/08/10/crows-are-surprisingly-good-at-making-tools-study-finds; Christian Rutz, Shoko Sugasawa, Jessica E. M. van der Wal, Barbara C. Klump, and James J. H. St. Clair, "Tool Bending in New Caledonian Crows," *Royal Society Open Science* (August 2016), http://rsos.royalsocietypublishing.org/content/royopensci/3/8/160439.full.pdf.

58 Andy Wright, "Pigheaded: How Smart are Swine?" Modern Farmer, March 10, 2014, https://modernfarmer.com/2014/03/pigheaded-smart-swine.

59 Laurent Keller and Élisabeth Gordon, *The Lives of Ants* (Oxford: Oxford University Press, 2010).

60 "The Bonds of Empathy: From Rats to Humans, Q&A with Jean Decety," Cognitive Neuroscience Society, www.cogneurosociety.org/bonds-of-empathy.

61 Karin Bruilliard, "New Study of Cats Significant in Its Rarity Compared with Dog Research," *Columbus Dispatch*, April 9, 2017, www.dispatch.com/news/20170409/new-study-of-cats-significant-in-its-rarity-compared-with-dog-research.

62 Jonathon Balcombe, *What a Fish Knows: The Inner Lives of Our Underwater Cousins* (London: Oneworld, 2016).

63 "Slime Mold Gives Insight into the Intelligence of Neuron-less Organisms," Phys.org, June 8, 2016, https://phys.org/news/2016-06-slime-mold-insight-intelligence-neuron-less.html.

64 Corey Charlton, "All Ground Beef Eaten in U.S. Contains Food Poisoning Bacteria: Study Reveals Dangers If Meat Is Not Properly Cooked," Daily Mail, August 26, 2015, www.dailymail.co.uk/news/article-3211443/All-ground-beef-eaten-U-S-contains-fecal-contamination-Study-reveals-dangers-poisoning-meat-not-properly-cooked.html; "Health and Safety," US Department of Agriculture, www.usda.gov/topics/health-and-safety.

65 "Food Safety for Pregnant Women," US Department of Agriculture, www.fda.gov/food/foodborneillnesscontaminants/peopleatrisk/ucm312704.htm#common.

66 "The Carbon Foodprint of Five Diets Compared," Shrink That Footprint, http://shrinkthatfootprint.com/food-carbon-footprint-diet; Peter Scarborough, Paul N. Appleby, Anja Mizdrak, Adam D. M. Briggs, Ruth C. Travis, Kathryn E. Bradbury, and Timothy J. Key, "Dietary Greenhouse Gas Emissions of Meat-Eaters, Fish-eaters, Vegetarians and Vegans in the UK," Climatic Change 125, no. 2 (July 2014): 179–192, https://link.springer.com/article/10.1007/s10584-014-1169-1/fulltext.html; David Pimentel and Marcia Pimental, "Sustainability of Meat-Based and Plant-Based Diets and the Environment," American Journal of Clinical Nutrition 78. no 3 (September 2003): 660S–663S, http://ajcn.nutrition.org/content/78/3/660S.full; "Facts on Animal Farming and the Environment," One Green Planet, www.onegreenplanet.org/animalsandnature/facts-on-animal-farming-and-the-environment; "Vegetarianism and the Environment. Why Going Meatless Is Important," Vegetarian Guide, https://michaelbluejay.com/veg/environment.html; "Our Future Our Food: Making a Difference with Every Bite: The Power of the Fork!" Earth Save International, 2006, www.earthsave.org/pdf/ofof2006.pdf; Janet Ranganathan and Richard Waite, "Sustainable Diets: What You Need to Know in 12 Charts," World Resources Institute, April 20, 2016, www.wri.org/blog/2016/04/sustainable-diets-what-you-need-know-12-charts; "The Facts," Cowspiracy.

67 "Meat Eater's Guide to Climate Change and Health," Environmental Working Group, 2011, http://static.ewg.org/reports/2011/meateaters/pdf/methodology_ewg_meat_eaters_guide_to_health_and_climate_2011.pdf; http://static.ewg.org/reports/2011/meateaters/pdf/methodology_ewg_meat_eaters_guide_to_health_and_climate_2011.pdf; Ranganathan and Waite, "Sustainable Diets: What You Need to Know in 12 Charts"; "How Much Have You Saved?" The Vegan Calculator, http://thevegancalculator.com/#calculator; Lillie Ogden, "The Environmental Impact of a Meat-Based Diet," Vegetarian Times, April 4, 2007, www.vegetariantimes.com/life-garden/the-environmental-impact-of-a-meat-based-diet.

68 Marco Springmann, H. Charles J. Godfray, Mike Raymer, and Peter Scarborough, "Analysis and Valuation of the Health and Climate Change

Cobenefit of Dietary Change," *PNAS* 113, no. 15 (April 2016): 4146–4151; "Plant-Based Diets Could Save Millions of Lives and Dramatically Cut Greenhouse Gas Emissions," Oxford Martin School, March 21, 2016, www.oxfordmartin.ox.ac.uk/news/201603_Plant_based_diets.

69 "New Bans on Plastic Bags May Help Protect Marine Life," Worldwatch Institute, www.worldwatch.org/node/5565.

70 "Questions and Answers About Palm Oil," Rainforest Rescue, www.rainforest-rescue.org/topics/palm-oil/questions-and-answers.

71 Michal Adaddy, "Palm Oil Could Kill Off Wild Orangutans in Just 10 Years," *Fortune*, August 22, 2016, fortune.com/2016/08/22/palm-oil-orangutan.

72 Adam Chandler, "Why Americans Lead the World in Food Waste," *Atlantic*, July 15, 2016, www.theatlantic.com/business/archive/2016/07/american-food-waste/491513; JoAnne Berkenkamp, "Imperfect Fruits and Vegetables: 15 Minutes of Fame or Lasting Paradigm Shift?" Natural Resources Defense Council, June 24, 2015, www.nrdc.org/experts/joanne-berkenkamp/imperfect-fruits-and-vegetables-15-minutes-fame-or-lasting-paradigm-shift.

73 "8 Things You Never Knew About Produce Stickers," *Morning Express with Robin Meade*, April 28, 2016, www.hlntv.com/shows/morning-express-robin-meade/articles/2014/01/15/8-things-you-never-knew-about-produce-stickers.

74 Jennifer Rude Klett, "Cost of Bulk vs. Packaged Foods," *Journal Sentinel*, January 31, 2017, www.jsonline.com/story/life/food/2017/01/31/cost-bulk-vs-packaged-foods/97090112.

75 "Defect Levels Handbook," US Food and Drug Administration, www.fda.gov/Food/GuidanceRegulation/GuidanceDocumentsRegulatoryInformation/SanitationTransportation/ucm056174.htm.

Give a Shit: In Your Closet

1 Ravi Dhar and Klaus Wertenbroch, "Consumer Choice Between Hedonic and Utilitarian Goods," *Journal of Marketing Research* 37 (February 2000): 60–71, http://faculty.som.yale.edu/ravidhar/documents/ConsumerChoicebetweenHedonicandUtilitarianGoods.pdf; Ran Kivetz and Yuhuang Zheng, "The Effects of Promotions on Hedonic versus Utilitarian Purchases," *Science Direct*, 27, no. 1 (January 2017): 59–68; Stuart Vise, *Going Broke: Why Americans Can't Hold on to Their Money* (Oxford: Oxford University Press, 2008); Jingyi Lu, Zhengyan Liu, and Zhe Fang, "Hedonic Products for You, Utilitarian Products for Me," *Judgment and Decision Making* 11, no. 4 (July 2016): 332–341, http://journal.sjdm.org/16/16428a/jdm16428a.pdf; Scott Rick and George Loewenstein, "The Role of Emotion in Economic Behavior," in *Handbook of Emotions*, 3rd ed., ed. Michael Lewis, Jeannete M. Haviland-Jones, and Lisa Feldman Barrett, 138–156 (New York: Guilford Press, 2010).

2 Shannon Whitehead, "5 Truths the Fast Fashion Industry Doesn't Want You to Know," *Huffington Post*, August 19, 2014, www.huffingtonpost.com/shannon-whitehead/5-truths-the-fast-fashion_b_5690575.html.

3 Scott Christian, "Fast Fashion Is Absolutely Destroying the Planet," *Esquire*, November 14, 2016; Alden Wicker, "Now We Know! Fashion Is the 5th Most Polluting Industry, Equal to Livestock," EcoCult, May 9, 2017, https://ecocult.com/now-know-fashion-5th-polluting-industry-equal-livestock.

4 Maxine Bédat and Michael Shank, "There Is a Major Climate Issue Hiding in Your Closet: Fast Fashion," *Fast Company*, November 11, 2016, www.fastcompany.com/3065532/there-is-a-major-climate-issue-hiding-in-your-closet-fast-fashion.

5 "Fast Fashion: What's the True Cost of a Bargain?" MIT Management Executive Education, https://executive.mit.edu/blog/fast-fashion-whats-the-true-cost-of-a-bargain#.WgUDoUxFyHm.

6 Alden Wicker, "Fast Fashion Is Creating an Environmental Crisis," *Newsweek*, September 1, 2016, www.newsweek.com/2016/09/09/old-clothes-fashion-waste-crisis-494824.html.

7 "Advancing Sustainable Materials Management: Facts and Figures," US Environmental Protection Agency, www.epa.gov/smm/advancing-sustainable-materials-management-facts-and-figures.

8 Elizabeth Kirk, "Recycling with Sole," Waste360, April 1, 2010, www.waste360.com/Recycling_And_Processing/shoe-recycling-201004.

9 "Child Labour," International Labour Organization, www.ilo.org/global/topics/child-labour/lang—en/index.htm.

10 "Tackling Child Labour in the Fashion Industry," Phys.org, June 13, 2017, https://phys.org/news/2017-06-tackling-child-labour-fashion-industry.html; Marc Bain, "'A Web of Terror, Insecurity, and a High Level of Vulnerability': H&M, Gap, and Walmart Are Accused of Widespread Worker Abuse," *Quartz*, May 31, 2016, https://qz.com/695763/a-web-of-terror-insecurity-and-a-high-level-of-vulnerability-hm-gap-and-walmart-are-accused-of-hundreds-of-acts-of-worker-abuse.

11 C&A Foundation, ICRW, Levi Strauss Foundation, and BSR, "Empowering Female Workers in the Industry: Three Areas for Business Action," June 2017, www.bsr.org/reports/BSR_Empowering_Female_Workers_in_the_Apparel_Industry.pdf; "In Bangladesh, Empowering and Employing Women in the Garments Sector," World Bank, February 7, 2017, www.worldbank.org/en/news/feature/2017/02/07/in-bangladesh-empowering-and-employing-women-in-the-garments-sector.

12 "Follow the Thread," Human Rights Watch, April 20, 2017, www.hrw.org/report/2017/04/20/follow-thread/need-supply-chain-transparency-garment-and-footwear-industry.

13 Elizabeth Segran, "The Real Story Behind Those Desperate Notes That Zara Workers Left in Clothes," *Fast Company*, November 6, 2017, www.fastcompany.com/40492215/the-real-story-behind-those-desperate-notes-that-zara-workers-left-in-clothes.

14 "Leather," US Legal, https://environmentallaw.uslegal.com/specific-issues/ leather; Justin Kenny and Larry C. Price, "Bangladesh's Leather Industry Exposes Workers and Children to Toxic Hazards," *PBS NewsHour*, March 30, 2017, http://pulitzercenter.org/reporting/bangladeshs-leather-industry-exposes-workers-and-children-toxic-hazards.

15 Scott Christian, "This Is Why Men Wear Only 13 Percent of Their Clothes," *Esquire*, September 10, 2015, www.esquire.com/style/mens-fashion/news/ a37832/a-study-finds-that-men-only-wear-13-percent-of-whats-in-their-closet; Barbara Brownie, "Why We Keep Clothes We Never Wear," *Guardian*, August 5, 2013, www.theguardian.com/fashion/costume-and-culture/2013/ aug/05/why-we-keep-clothes-never-wear; Kathryn Vasel, "You're Organizing Your Closet All Wrong," *CNN Money*, November 21, 2014, http://money.cnn. com/2014/1½1/luxury/organize-closet-tips/index.html.

16 Chris Tyree and Dan Morrison, "Invisibles," https://orbmedia.org/stories/ Invisibles_plastics.

17 Stephanie Rosenblum, "Fashion Tries on Zero Waste Design," *New York Times*, August 13, 2010, www.nytimes.com/2010/08/15/fashion/15waste.html?_r=0.

18 Laura Moss, "Massive Investigation Finds So-Called Fake Fur May Be Real," *Business Insider*, January 31, 2014, www.businessinsider.com/humane-society-finds-real-fur-mislabeled-as-faux-2014-1.

Give a Shit: In the Mirror

1 "Safety Testing and Health Research for the 21st Century," Humane Society International, hsi.org/campaigns/end_animal_testing.

2 "In Testing," NEAVS, www.neavs.org/alternatives/in-testing.

3 Wayne Pacelle, "HSUS Calls on L'Oréal to Embrace a Global Ban on Animal Testing for Cosmetics," A Humane Nation, September 19, 2017, https://blog. humanesociety.org/wayne/2017/09/hsus-calls-loreal-embrace-global-ban-animal-testing-cosmetics.html.

4 Jessica Chia, "The 8 Weirdest Animal Ingredients in Your Beauty Products," *Prevention*, March 28, 2014, www.prevention.com/beauty/natural-beauty/the-8-weirdest-animal-ingredients-in-your-beauty-products.

5 "Fighting Animal Testing," Lush, www.lushusa.com/about-animal-introduction. html.

6 "'Cruelty Free'/'Not Tested on Animals'," US Food and Drug Administration, www.fda.gov/cosmetics/labeling/claims/ucm2005202.htm.

7 Adina Grigore, *Skin Cleanse: The Simple, All-Natural Program for Clear, Calm, Happy Skin* (New York: HarperCollins, 2018), 131.

8 "What Does Our Symbol Mean?" Soil Association, www.soilassociation.org/ organic-living/beauty-wellbeing/what-does-our-symbol-mean.

9 "Personal Care Product Certification," Oregon Tilth, https://tilth.org/certification/forms/personal-care-products.

10 Jareen Imam, "8 Trillion Microbeads Pollute U.S. Aquatic Habitats Daily," CNN, October 6, 2015, www.cnn.com/2015/09/19/us/8-trillion-microbeads-pollute-water-daily-irpt/index.html.

11 Harsharnjit S. Gill, "Probiotics to Enhance Anti-Infective Defences in the Gastrointestinal Tract," *Best Practice & Research Clinical Gastroenterology* 17, no. 5 (2003): 755–773.

12 "Antibacterial Soap? You Can Skip It, Use Plain Soap and Water," US Food and Drug Administration, www.fda.gov/ForConsumers/ConsumerUpdates/ucm378393.htm; Allison E. Aiello, Elaine L. Larson, and Stuart B. Levy, "Consumer Antibacterial Soaps: Effective or Just Risky?" *Clinical Infectious Diseases* 45, no. S2 (September 2007): S137–S147.

13 Coco Ballantyne, "Strange but True: Antibacterial Products May Do More Harm Than Good," *Scientific American*, June 7, 2007, www.scientificamerican.com/article/strange-but-true-antibacterial-products-may-do-more-harm-than-good.

14 Antonia M. Calafat, Xiaoyun Ye, Lee-Yang Wong, John A. Reidy, and Larry L. Needham, "Urinary Concentrations of Triclosan in the U.S. Population: 2003–2004," *Environmental Health Perspectives* 116, no. 3 (March 2008): 303–307.

15 Tammy E. Stoker, Emily K. Gibson, and Leah M. Zorrilla, "Triclosan Exposure Modulates Estrogen-Dependent Responses in the Female Wistar Rat," *Toxicological Sciences* 117, no. 1 (September 2010): 45–53; "5 Things to Know About Triclosan," US Food and Drug Administration, www.fda.gov/ForConsumers/ConsumerUpdates/ucm205999.htm; S. H. Sicherer and D. Y. Leung, "Advances in Allergic Skin Disease, Anaphylaxis, and Hypersensitivity Reactions to Foods, Drugs, and Insects in 2012," *Journal of Allergy and Clinical Immunology* 131, no. 1 (January 2013): 55–66.

Give a Shit: In the Wild

1 "Municipal Solid Waste," US Environmental Protection Agency.

2 "Goals & Progress: Reusable Cups," Starbucks, www.starbucks.com/responsibility/global-report/environmental-stewardship/reusable-cups.

3 PepsiCo Recycling, Keep America Beautiful and CBRE, "Recycling at Work," April 2015, www.kab.org/sites/default/files/RecyclingatWork_Workplace_Recycling_Research_Final_Report_April2015.pdf.

4 "Sustainability's Strategic Worth: McKinsey Global Survey Results," McKinsey & Company, June 2014, www.mckinsey.com/business-functions/sustainability-and-resource-productivity/our-insights/sustainabilitys-strategic-worth-mckinsey-global-survey-results; "Report Shows a Third of Consumers Prefer Sustainable Brands," Unilever, May 1, 2017, www.unilever.com/news/Press-releases/2017/report-shows-a-third-of-consumers-prefer-sustainable-brands.html.

5 "Sustainability's Strategic Worth."

6 "Can Birth Control Hormones Be Filtered from the Water Supply?" *Scientific American*, www.scientificamerican.com/article/birth-control-in-water-supply.

7 "About Paragard," Paragard, http://paragard.com/about-paragard.aspx.

8 Diana Rodriguez, "The Truth About the Rhythm Method," *Everyday Health*, www.everydayhealth.com/sexual-health/rhythm-method.aspx.

9 Damian Carrington, "Want to Fight Climate Change? Have Fewer Kids," *Guardian*, July 12, 2017, www.theguardian.com/environment/2017/jul/12/want-to-fight-climate-change-have-fewer-children; Seth Wynes and Kimberly A. Nicholas, "The Climate Mitigation Gap: Education and Government Recommendations Miss the Most Effective Individual Actions," *Environmental Research Letters* 12, no. 7 (July 2017); Tori Whitley, "Want to Slow Global Warming? Researchers Look to Family Planning," *Morning Edition*, NPR, July 18, 2017, www.npr.org/2017/07/19/537954372/want-to-slow-global-warming-researchers-look-to-family-planning.

10 United Nations, "World Population Prospects," 2015, https://esa.un.org/unpd/wpp/Publications/Files/Key_Findings_WPP_2015.pdf.

11 IPCC, "Climate Change 2014," www.ipcc.ch/report/ar5/syr.

12 Rebecca Winthrop and Homi Kharas, "Want to Save the Planet? Invest in Girls' Education," Brookings Institution, March 3, 2016, www.brookings.edu/opinions/want-to-save-the-planet-invest-in-girls-education.

13 "AFCARS Report #23," Children's Bureau, June 30, 2016, www.acf.hhs.gov/cb/resource/afcars-report-23; Michael Winerip, "Out of Foster Care, Into College," *New York Times*, October 30, 2013, www.nytimes.com/2013/11/03/education/edlife/extra-support-can-make-all-the-difference-for-foster-youth.html.

14 "Statistics on Youth Aging Out of Foster Care," National CASA, http://nc.casaforchildren.org/files/secure/community/programs/Training/2016%20Pilot/Statistics%20on%20Youth%20Aging%20Out%20of%20Foster%20Care.PDF.

15 "A Look at Wedding Industry Waste + Eco-Friendly Wedding Tips," Botanical Paperworks, www.botanicalpaperworks.com/blog/read,article/718/a-look-at-wedding-industry-waste-eco-friendly-wedding-tips; Carter Reum, "The Secret Waste That Weddings Leave Behind," *Huffington Post*, April 20, 2012, www.huffingtonpost.com/carter-reum/the-secret-waste-that-weddings-leave_b_1439118.html; Danielle Calhoun, "10 Ways to Waste Less on Your Wedding Day!" Black Sheep Bride, https://blacksheepbride.com/10-ways-to-waste-less-on-your-wedding-day.

16 "How Far Does Your Food Travel to Get to Your Plate?" CUESA, https://

cuesa.org/learn/how-far-does-your-food-travel-get-your-plate.

17 Rebecca Smithers, "For Richer, for Poorer . . . a Tenth of All Wedding Food Is Thrown Away," *Guardian*, July 28, 2017, www.theguardian.com/environment/2017/jul/28/tenth-of-wedding-food-thrown-away.

18 "Impacts on Wildlife & the Environment: Balloons Kill Wildlife," Ballons Blow . . . Don't Let Them Go!, https://balloonsblow.org/impacts-on-wildlife-and-environment.

19 "Household, Individual, and Vehicle Characteristics," Bureau of Transportation Statistics, www.rita.dot.gov/bts/sites/rita.dot.gov.bts/files/publications/highlights_of_the_2001_national_household_travel_survey/html/section_01.html; "Sources of Greenhouse Gas Emissions," US Environmental Protection Agency, www.epa.gov/ghgemissions/sources-greenhouse-gas-emissions; "Cars Emissions & Global Warming," Union of Concerned Scientists, www.ucsusa.org/clean-vehicles/car-emissions-and-global-warming#.WgUWKUxFyHl.

20 "Overweight and Obesity Statistics," National Institute of Diabetes and Digestive and Kidney Diseases, www.niddk.nih.gov/health-information/health-statistics/overweight-obesity.

21 Tom Anderson, "Commuters Waste a Full Week in Traffic Each Year," CNBC, August 9, 2016, www.cnbc.com/2016/08/09/commuters-waste-a-full-week-in-traffic-each-year.html.

22 Sarah Knapton, " How to Save the Planet: Cut Holidays, Sell the Car and Don't Have as Many Children, Say Scientists," *Telegraph*, July 12, 2017, www.telegraph.co.uk/science/2017/07/11/save-planet-cut-holidays-sell-car-dont-have-many-children-say.

23 "What Is the Largest Metro System in the World?" CityMetric, September 5, 2015, www.citymetric.com/transport/what-largest-metro-system-world-1361; "List of Bicycle-Sharing Systems," Wikipedia, https://en.wikipedia.org/wiki/List_of_bicycle-sharing_systems.

24 "Facts & Figures," Air Transport Action Group, www.atag.org/facts-and-figures.html; Natasha Geiling, "Can Eco-Conscious Travelers Do Anything to Fly Green?" *Smithsonian*, August 11, 2014, www.smithsonianmag.com/travel/if-you-travel-and-care-about-environment-you-should-buy-carbon-offsets-180952222/.

25 "Planes Utilize Most Fuel During Takeoff," Worldwatch Institute, www.worldwatch.org/planes-utilize-most-fuel-during-takeoff.

26 Heinrich Bofinger and Jon Strand, "Calculating the Carbon Footprint from Different Classes of Air Travel," World Bank, May 2013, http://documents.worldbank.org/curated/en/141851468168853188/pdf/WPS6471.pdf.

27 Rachel Nuwer, "Reusing Hotel Towels Actually Does Make a Difference," *Smithsonian*, February 25, 2014, www.smithsonianmag.com/smart-news/reusing-hotel-towels-actually-does-make-difference-180949890.

28 Parija Kavilanz, "Dreaming of a Trashy Christmas," CNN Money, December 17, 2010, http://money.cnn.com/2010/12/16/news/economy/holiday_trash/index.htm; Nicki Lisa Cole, "Christmas: What We Do, How We Spend, and Why It Matters," ThoughtCo., March 2, 2017, www.thoughtco.com/christmas-what-we-do-how-we-spend-and-why-it-matters-3026192; Eleanor Goldberg, "You Won't Believe How Much Crap Americans Throw Out Over the Holidays," *Huffington Post*, December 20, 2016, www.huffingtonpost.com/entry/christmas-trash-waste_us_5852d4f7e4b0c05ff31ffeab; "Reduce, Recycle, Reuse," US Environmental Protection Agency, www3.epa.gov/region9/waste/recycling.

29 "Global Warming: Give the Gift of Green," Oprah.com, www.oprah.com/oprahshow/holiday-ecology/2; "Facts About Paper and Paper Waste," iD2 Communications, www.id2.ca/downloads/eco-design-paper-facts.pdf; "Frequently Asked Questions: Holiday Waste Prevention," Stanford University, https://lbre.stanford.edu/pssistanford-recycling/frequently-asked-questions/frequently-asked-questions-holiday-waste-prevention.

30 "Turkeys Used for Food," PETA, www.peta.org/issues/animals-used-for-food/factory-farming/turkeys.

31 "Frequently Asked Questions: Holiday Waste Prevention," Stanford University; "How to Recycle Paper," Earth911, earth911.com/recycling-guide/how-to-recycle-paper.

32 Marie Carter, "Why Having a Pet Is Good for Your Health," *Independent*, December 31, 2015, www.independent.co.uk/life-style/health-and-families/features/how-having-a-pet-can-make-us-healthier-a6792126.html.

33 "Pet Statistics," ASPCA, www.aspca.org/animal-homelessness/shelter-intake-and-surrender/pet-statistics.

Sidebar Endnotes

Introduction

i "Overview of Greenhouse Gasses," US Environmental Protection Agency, www.epa.gov/ghgemissions/overview-greenhouse-gases.

ii "Great Pacific Garbage Patch," Wikipedia, https://en.wikipedia.org/wiki/Great_Pacific_garbage_patch.

Give a Shit: In Your Home

i U.S. and World Population Clock, Census.gov, www.census.gov/popclock; "What Is the United States' Share of World Energy Consumption?" Frequently Asked Questions, US Energy Information Administration, www.eia.gov/tools/faqs/faq.php?id=87&t=1; Maya Wei-Haas, "How America Stacks Up When It Comes to Greenhouse Gas Emissions," *Smithsonian magazine*, June 2, 20017, www.smithsonianmag.com/smart-news/how-America-stacks-up-greenhouse-gas-emissions-180963560; "Inventory of U.S. Greenhouse Gas Emissions and Sinks: 1990–2015," Greenhouse Gas Emissions, US Environmental Protections Agency, www.epa.gov/ghgemissions/inventory-us-greenhouse-gas-emissions-and-sinks-1990-2015; "Population and Energy Consumption," World Population Balance, www.worldpopulationbalance.org/population_energy.

ii "How Much Energy Is Consumed in U.S. Residential and Commercial Buildings?" Frequently Asked Questions, US Energy Information Administration, www.worldpopulationbalance.org/population_energy; "Consumption and Efficiency," US Energy Information Administration, www.eia.gov/consumption; "Average Household Electricity Use Around the World," Shrink That Footprint, http://shrinkthatfootprint.com/average-household-electricity-consumption Global Energy Use Statistics; Lela Nargi, "Think Your Household Is Sustainable? Think Again," *Sierra*, January 27, 2017, www.sierraclub.org/sierra/green-life/think-your-household-sustainable-think-again.

iii "How Much Energy Is Consumed in U.S. Residential and Commercial Buildings?"; "Consumption and Efficiency"; Tariq Khokhar, "Chart: Over 1 Billion People Had No Access to Electricity in 2014," The Data Blog, World Bank, April 3, 2017, https://blogs.worldbank.org/opendata/chart-over-1-billion-people-had-no-access-electricity-2014; Nargi, "Think Your Household Is Sustainable? Think Again."

iv Roni A. Neff, Marie L. Spiker, Patricia L. Truant, "Wasted Food: U.S. Consumers' Reported Awareness, Attitudes, and Behaviors," *PLOS One* 10, no. 6 (June 10, 2015), https://doi.org/10.1371/journal.pone.0127881; "Don't Waste, Donate: Enhancing Food Donations Through Federal Policy, Harvard Food Law and Policy Center, National Resources Defense Council, March

2017, https://drive.google.com/viewerng/viewer?url=http://archive.azcentral.
com/persistent/icimages/thingstodo/Dont-Waste-Donate_-March-2017.
pdf?from%3Dglobal; Danyi Qi and Brian E. Roe, "Household Food Waste:
Multivariate Regression and Principal Components Analyses of Awareness
and Attitudes Among U.S. Consumers," *PLOS One* 11, no. 7 (July 21, 2016),
https://doi.org/10.1371/journal.pone.0159250; Jonathan Bloom, "In United
States, There's a Lot of Food Being Wasted," *Washington Post*, June 20, 2012,
www.washingtonpost.com/in-united-states-theres-a-lot-of-food-being-
wasted/2012/06/19/gJQAmk9JoV_story.html?utm_term=.080c1187cf6b.

v Viviana Solorzano and Andrew Edwards, "Memo: Executive Summary
Report—Composting," Harris Interactive, December 27, 2013, www.recycle.
cc/2013-1227NW&RA_composting_survey_executive_summary_010814.
pdfCompost Study Memo.

vi "2015 Characteristics of New Housing," US Department of Housing and
Urban Development and US Department of Commerce: Characteristics of
New Housing, 2015, www.census.gov/construction/chars/pdf/c25ann2015.
pdf; Self Storage Industry Specifics, Statistic Brain, www.statisticbrain.com/
self-storage-industry-statistics; Mary MacVean, " For Many People, Gathering
Possessions Is Just the Stuff of Life," *Los Angeles Times*, March 21, 2014, http://
articles.latimes.com/2014/mar/21/health/la-he-keeping-stuff-20140322.

vii "Car Ownership in U.S. Cities Map," Governing, www.governing.com/
gov-data/car-ownership-numbers-of-vehicles-by-city-map.html; "How
Many Alternative Fuel and Hybrid Vehicles Are There in the United States?"
Frequently Asked Questions, US Energy Information Administration, www.eia.
gov/tools/faqs/faq.php?id=93&t=4.

viii Drew Desilver, "Perceptions and Realities of Recycling Vary Widely from
Place to Place," Pew Research Center, October 7, 2106, www.pewresearch.
org/fact-tank/2016/10/07/perceptions-and-realities-of-recycling-vary-widely-
from-place-to-place.

ix David J. Nowak, Nathaniel Appleton, Alexis Ellis, and Eric Greenfield,
"Residential Building Energy Conservations and Avoided Power Plant Emissions
by Urban and Community Trees in the United States," *Urban Forestry and
Urban Greening* 21, (2017): 158–165, https://www.fs.fed.us/nrs/pubs/jrnl/2017/
nrs_2017_nowak_001.pdf.

x "Benefit of Trees," Arbor Day Foundation, www.arborday.org/trees/
benefits.cfm; "Plant Trees to Save Energy and Grow Value," Houselogic, www.
houselogic.com/by-room/yard-patio/plant-trees-save-energy-grow-value.

xi Patrick Sisson, "In Nation of Hoarders, Self-Storage Spots Outnumber
McDonald's," Curbed, April 20, 2015, www.curbed.com/2015/4/20/9969068/
in-nation-of-hoarders-self-storage-spots-outnumber-mcdonalds; Suzy
Strutner, "American Has More Self-Storage Facilities Than McDonald's,

Because Apparently We're All Hoarders, *Huffington Post*, April 21, 2015, www. huffingtonpost.com/2015/04/21/self-storage-mcdonalds_n_7107822.html.

xii Mark Huffman, "Seniors Bombarded with Direct Mail Often Write Many Checks," Consumer Affairs, June 26, 2013, www.consumeraffairs.com/news/ seniors-bombarded-with-direct-mail-often-write-many-checks-062613.html.

xiii "Winter Warmers: The Cold Facts About Down, Angora and Wool," Animals Australia, www.animalsaustralia.org/features/winter-warmers-cold-facts- about-down-wool-angora.php.

xiv Emma Miller, "6 Easy Ways to Go Green in Your Office, Green Future, https://greenfuture.io/sustainable-living/environmentally-sustainable- practices-in-the-workplace; Ben, "The Problem with Plastic Pens . . . ," OpenIdeo, June 11, 2017, https://challenges.openideo.com/challenge/ circular-design/research/the-problem-with-plastic-pens; "The Environmental Consumer's Handbook," US Environmental Protection Agency, http://bit. ly/2AkMzoy; "Cutting Trash Down to Size," *New York Times*, October 11, 1988, www.nytimes.com/1988/10/11/opinion/cutting-trash-down-to-size.html.

xv Jason Slotkin, "Behold the Fatberg: London's 130-Ton, 'Rock-Solid' Sewer Blockage," *The Two-Way*, NPR, September 12, 2017, www.npr.org/sections/ thetwo-way/2017/09/12/550465000/behold-the-fatberg-london-s-130-ton- rock-solid-sewer-blockage.   .

xvi "How to Reduce Your Paper Towel Use," The Paperless Project, www. thepaperlessproject.com/how-to-reduce-your-paper-towel-use.

Give a Shit: In the Kitchen

i "Fish and Other Sea Animals Used for Food," PETA, www.peta.org/issues/ animals-used-for-food/factory-farming/fish.

ii Zak Smith, Margaretmary Gilroy, Matthew Eisenson, Erin Schnettler, and Stephanie, Stefanski, "Net Loss: The Killing of Marine Mammals in Foreign Fisheries," NRDC Report, January 2014, www.nrdc.org/sites/default/files/ mammals-foreign-fisheries-report.pdf; Boris Worm, Brendal Davis, Lisa Kettemer, Christine A. Ward-Paige, Demian Chapman, Michael R. Heithaus, Steven T. Kessel et al., "Global Catches, Exploitation Rates, and Rebuilding Options for Sharks," *Marine Policy* 40 (2013): 194–204, wormlab.biology.dal. ca/publication/view/worm-etal-2013-global-catches-exploitation-rates-and- rebuilding-options-for-sharks; Dan Stone, "100 Million Sharks Killed Every Year, Study Show on Eve of International Conference on Shark Protection." *National Geographic*, Ocean Views, March 1, 2013, voices.nationalgeographic. org/2013/03/01/100-million-sharks-killed-every-year-study-shows-on-eve-of- international-conference-on-shark-protection.

iii Harish, "How Many Animals Does a Vegetarian Save?" Counting Animals,

February 6, 2012, http://countinganimals.com/how-many-animals-does-a-vegetarian-save.

iv Dnews, "Oceans' Fish Could Disappear by 2050," Seeker, May 17, 2010, www.seeker.com/oceans-fish-could-disappear-by-2050-1765058733.html; Brian Merchant, "By 2100, "Earth Will Have an Entirely Different Ocean," Motherboard, August 13, 2015, https://motherboard.vice.com/en_us/article/bmjqvz/by-2100-everything-you-know-about-the-ocean-will-be-wrong; Emily Moran Barwick, "How Many Animals Do We Kill Every Year?" Bite Size Vegan, May 27, 2015, http://bitesizevegan.com/ethics-and-morality/quantifying-suffering-cruelty-by-the-numbers.

v "Executive Summary," EWG, www.ewg.org/foodnews/summary.php#.Wh7RekxFw0Q.

vi Pamela Riemenschneider, "2017 'Dirty Dozen' and 'Clean 15' Lists Revealed," Produce Retailer, March 9, 2017, www.produceretailer.com/article/news-article/2017-dirty-dozen-and-clean-15-lists-released.

Give a Shit: In the Mirror

i "Fact Sheet: Cosmetic Testing," Humane Society of the United States, www.humanesociety.org/issues/cosmetic_testing/qa/questions_answers.html.

ii "8 Products You Own That Are Tested on Animals," Business Insurance Quotes, www.businessinsurance.org/8-products-you-own-that-are-tested-on-animals; Jomo Merritt, "20 Everyday Products You Had No Clue Are Tested on Animals," The Clever, February 13, 2017, www.theclever.com/20-everyday-products-you-had-no-clue-are-tested-on-animals.

iii Pacelle, "HSUS Calls on L'Oréal to Embrace a Global Ban on Animal Testing for Cosmetics"; Sophia Yan, "In China, Big Cosmetics Firms Are Selling Products Tested on Animals," CNBC, April 19, 2017, www.cnbc.com/2017/04/19/in-china-big-cosmetics-firms-are-selling-products-tested-on-animals.html.

iv Loren Berlin, "Burt's Bees, Tom's of Maine Owned by Fortune 500 Companies," *Huffington Post*, April 20, 2012, www.huffingtonpost.com/2012/04/20/burts-bees-toms-of-maine-green-products_n_1438019.html.

v Carol Potera, "Indoor Air Quality: Scented Products Emit a Bouquet of VOCs," *Environmental Health Perspectives* 119, no. 1 (January 2011): A16.

vi "Air Fresheners Can Make Mothers and Babies Ill," University of Bristol, October 19, 2004, www.bristol.ac.uk/alspac/news/2004/75.html.

vii Rachel Bolton, "Menstrual Cups: Use Them. Period," *Odyssey*, November 17, 2015, www.theodysseyonline.com/menstrual-cups-period.

viii Jessica Kane, "Here's How Much a Woman's Period Will Cost Her Over a Lifetime," *Huffington Post*, May 18, 2015, www.huffingtonpost.com/2015/05/18/period-cost-lifetime_n_7258780.html.

Give a Shit: In the Wild

i "Bottled Water Facts," Ban the Bottle, www.banthebottle.net/bottled-water-facts.

ii "The Be Straw Free Campaign," NPS Commercial Services, www.nps.gov/commercialservices/greenline_straw_free.htm.

iii Chris Wilcox, Erik van Sebille, and Britta Denise Hardesty, "Threat of Plastic Pollution to Seabirds Is Global, Pervasive, and Increasing," *PNAS* 112, no. 38 (September 2015): 11899–11904; Qamar Schuyler, Britta Denise Hardesty, Chris Wilcox, and Kathy Townsend, "Global Analysis of Anthropogenic Debris Ingestion by Sea Turtles," *Conservation Biology* (August 2013): 1–11.

iv "School Waste Study," Minnesota Pollution Control Agency, www.pca.state.mn.us/waste/school-waste-study; "MPS by the Numbers," Minneapolis Public Schools," www.mpls.k12.mn.us/by_the_numbers.

v "Can Dogs Stay Healthy on a Vegetarian Diet?" PetMD, www.petmd.com/blogs/nutritionnuggets/jcoates/2014/jan/can-dogs-stay-healthy-on-a-vegetarian-diet-31188.

Index

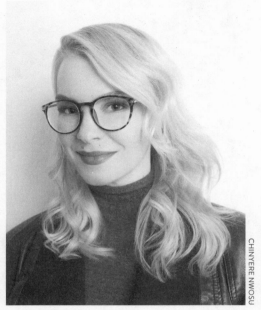

CHINYERE NWOSU

About the Author

Ashlee Piper is a political strategist turned eco-lifestyle journalist and TV personality. She's a regular contributor to Refinery29, *Women's Health*, ABC, CBS, and *Glamour*, among others. Piper holds a BA from Brown University and an MSc from the University of Oxford, UK. She lives in Chicago with her shelter dog, Banjo. You can learn more at www.ashleepiper.com.